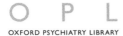

O P L
OXFORD PSYCHIATRY LIBRARY

Personality Disorder

T0177742

O P L
OXFORD PSYCHIATRY LIBRARY

Personality Disorder

Giles Newton-Howes

Senior Lecturer, Department of Psychological Medicine
Wellington School of Medicine
Otago University
New Zealand

Honorary Senior Lecturer, Department of Psychological Medicine
Imperial College
England

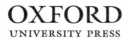

OXFORD
UNIVERSITY PRESS

OXFORD
UNIVERSITY PRESS

Great Clarendon Street, Oxford, OX2 6DP,
United Kingdom

Oxford University Press is a department of the University of Oxford.
It furthers the University's objective of excellence in research, scholarship,
and education by publishing worldwide. Oxford is a registered trade mark of
Oxford University Press in the UK and in certain other countries

Published in the United States of America by Oxford University Press
198 Madison Avenue, New York, NY 10016, United States of America

British Library Cataloguing in Publication Data
Data available

Library of Congress Control Number: 2014947262

ISBN 978–0–19–968838–8

Printed and bound in Great Britain by
Clays Ltd, St Ives plc

Contents

Foreword

Personality disorder is big. It is big in terms of its size (with one in ten people suffering from its impact), big in its impact on general functioning and quality of life, big in its propensity to create other mental and sometimes physical disorders, and big in terms of its cost to society. Dr Newton-Howes illustrates this beautifully in the comprehensive text you now hold. This pocketbook is written in straightforward language with excellent case examples from clinical practice, and it presents good empirical evidence in a subject area that until recently has been a minefield of speculation and dogma. As a guide to comprehensive understanding of people with mental distress of any sort, I could not recommend a better guide.

Professor Peter Tyrer

Preface

No field stands still. This is no truer than in the area of personality disorder where huge advances have been made in our understanding of assessment, diagnosis, and management. Along with this has come increasing recognition of the important place personality disorder has in psychiatric care. It is timely, therefore, to have a handbook for clinicians to use as a ready resource when they suspect the patient they are seeing may have personality pathology. If the clinician is a psychiatrist in secondary care services, prevalence alone suggests they are probably right. This highlights the need to consider the impact of personality in every patient reviewed. Although experts disagree about many aspects of personality disorder and a number of elements found within this book are potentially open to debate, the field has reached the point where identification has clinical utility. By keeping a focus on the most relevant aspects of personality pathology, clinicians can have confidence in their day-to-day work.

This book is designed to help clinicians in the understanding of personality and personality disorder as clinically useful constructs. It is divided into three broad sections. Chapter 1–3 provides a basic understanding of personality in terms of its development, current understanding, and its place in psychiatry. The focus is on clinical utility rather than unpacking the dense (and often confusing) literature that surrounds our psychological make-up, both normal and abnormal. Chapters 4–8 focuses closely on personality disorder as it presents in a clinical setting and is described by ICD-10 and DSM-5. For all their controversy these remain the classification systems most in use. Finally, the principles of management are outlined in Chapter 9–13, with a closer focus on the pharmacological, psychotherapeutic, and social interventions with an evidence base. The book concludes with a chapter on personality disorder as it presents in other mental state disorders. This book seeks to balance utility, evidence, and information for use in everyday practice.

Abbreviations

ADHD	attention deficit hyperactivity disorder
ASPD	antisocial personality disorder
BPAD	bipolar affective disorder
BPD	borderline personality disorder
CAT	cognitive analytical therapy
CBT-pd	cognitive behavioural therapy for personality disorder
DBT	dialectical behaviour therapy
DBT-S	dialectical behaviour therapy for substance abuse
DFST	dual-focus schema therapy
DPD	dependant personality disorder
DSM	Diagnostic and Statistical Manual
ED	emergency department
GAF	global assessment of functioning
HPD	histrionic personality disorder
ICD	International Classification of Disease
MBT	mentalization-based treatment
MSD	mental state disorder
NESARC	National Epidemiologic Survey on Alcohol and Related Conditions
NPD	narcissistic personality disorder
NSSI	non-suicidal self-injury
OCPD	obsessive–compulsive personality disorder
PD	personality disorder
PD-NOS	personality disorder 'Not Otherwise Specified'
PET	Positron emission tomography
PPD	paranoid personality disorder
ScPD	schizotypal personality disorder
SGA	second-generation antipsychotic
SFT	schema-focused therapy
SPD	schizoid personality disorder
SSRI	selective serotonin re-uptake inhibitors
STEPPS	systems training for emotional predictability and problem solving

SUD	substance disorder
TAU	treatment as usual
TC	therapeutic communities
TFP	transference-focused psychotherapy

Chapter 1

Introduction to personality disorder

The conceptualization and management of personality problems and their subsequent disorders is one of the most challenging areas in psychiatry. There is a fundamental need to be able to understand the psychological profile of every individual because it is through the landscape of a person's unique quirks and character traits that mental state disorder is manifested. It can also be the patient's personality itself that poses a problem to both them and others in society. Identifying this provides the opportunity to bring about positive change. Not only are there significant challenges in the diagnosis of personality disorder, but also this disorder has traditionally been considered 'untreatable', a grab-bag of symptoms falling outside the domain of mental health professionals. This has meant that teaching and research in personality disorder has been left behind that of many of the mental state disorders. Increasingly, however, the need to identify, diagnose, and manage personality problems is recognized as an issue for all clinicians involved in mental health, from primary care physicians to specialist personality disorder teams. This is increasingly recognized clinically and is reflected in the referral criteria of many psychiatric services. Managing presentations such as Ms ML proactively (see case vignette Ms ML) can lead to long-term positive change for the individual, reduced use of health services, and positive benefits for society.

In 1980, the American Psychiatric Association separated personality disorder from mental state disorder, placing it onto a separate axis, Axis II, in its multi-axial diagnostic system. From this stemmed a sharp rise in the time, energy, and resource spent on understanding personality problems, something that is reflected in the growth of the literature on the subject (Figure 1.1). From a clinical perspective, this translated into changes in the status of personality pathology in psychiatry. An example of this is the development of bio-psychosocial interventions aimed at addressing personality diathesis. From this emerging evidence there are now management strategies that may offer real benefits to patients with personality disorder in a similar manner to those offered for other psychiatric disorders. This is most true of borderline personality disorder (BPD), the diagnosis most commonly investigated. Many of the strategies trialled for BPD may have clinical implications in the management of other personality domains, and many of the individual elements of management can be extrapolated to treat other disorders. It is also increasingly clear that issues such as severity of personality difficulties are important.

As clinical diagnosis and recognition have evolved, the need to divide personality disorder from mental state disorder by placing it on a separate axis has become increasingly unnecessary. DSM-5 recognizes this and no longer uses the multi-axial system. Personality disorder has always been classified with other mental disorders in the ICD system. In Part III of DSM-5 a dimensional trait- and severity-based diagnostic system is presented. This is potentially a major shift towards a model of diagnosis closer to the structure of personality as it is understood and it makes allowances for the issue of severity. There is

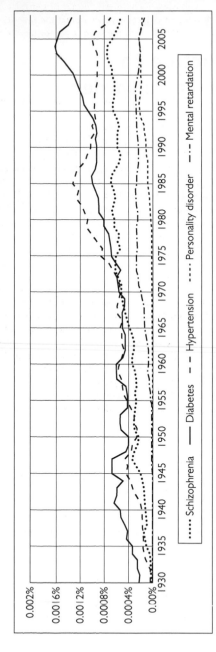

Figure 1.1 Ngram of the increase in the prevalence of the term 'personality disorder' in all books compared to other diagnostic terms, 1930–2008.

some indication that this may be the model used in future iterations of the ICD classification system. As becomes obvious when considering a case of personality disorder such as Ms ML, the most clinically relevant aspects revolve around the severity of psychopathology and non-suicidal self-injury (NSSI), with the specific personality disorder label of less immediate relevance.

Case vignette—Ms ML

Ms ML was a 22-year-old woman who presented to the emergency department (ED) with her girlfriend in the evening. Following an argument, she had cut her right forearm. She explained she had been arguing with her partner and the argument got out of hand. She had been unable to cope and when her partner told her to 'go do it' she decided that cutting herself would show she was willing to end her life if her partner did not love her. She confessed to being in a difficult relationship and said she was often low in mood with little energy or concentration during the day. She agreed she slept poorly and ate in an erratic fashion but did not lose weight. Her future goals included finding work and getting married to her partner of three months. She denied symptoms suggestive of mania or psychosis although she reported often hearing 'a voice in my head' telling her to kill herself. She agreed that she thought about dying on at least a weekly basis but did not think she had ever tried to commit suicide. She denied wanting to die at the interview in the ED. She admitted to an overdose of 20 tablets of paracetamol approximately three months earlier, 'to make it all go away', and to cutting on both arms and legs to help her when distressed. The was no history of major medical problems and no prior presentation to psychiatric services although Ms ML had presented to the emergency room six times in the last eight months with cuts and complaints of pain requiring opiate analgesia. She denied significant alcohol use or any illicit drug use. She was vague about her family history and would not answer questions about her personal life other than to say she had a part-time job, a partner with whom she lived, and 'amazing friends'. Ms ML lived in rented accommodation without family nearby. She stated she was keen to return home that evening, felt she would be fine because her partner was with her, and did not want any further assistance. Her laceration required exploration to ensure no tendon damage and suturing.

Ms ML presents with a probable personality disorder and her differential diagnosis includes a depressive disorder and possibly an opiate-use disorder. Her immediate risks are low; however, she describes a gradual increase in the severity of self-harm and one potentially fatal event (the overdose). She is likely, therefore to benefit from further discussion about an extended assessment to clarify her diagnosis and to consider what treatment options are available to her. She is very unlikely to meet the requirements for forcible treatment under the Mental Health Act and doing so would potentially lead to significant longer-term harm. Ideally, engaging her in a discussion as to the probable diagnosis and possible treatment options may help Ms ML to recognize that she has difficulties in understanding herself and her relationships with others, and there may be ways to improve this. Preferably this would be done the next morning on the surgical ward but failing this, it would be worth doing in the ED despite the late hour.

Key references

American Psychiatric Association. DSM-IV. –Arlington, VA: American Psychiatric Publishing, Inc., 2000.

Hopwood, C. J., Malone, J. C., Ansell, E. B., Sanislow, C. A., Grilo, C. M., Pinto, A., Markowitz, J. C., Shea, M. T., Skodol, A. E., Gunderson, J. G., Zanarini, M. C., Morey, L. C. Personality Assessment in DSM-5: Empirical support for rating Severity, Style, and Traits. *Journal of Personality Disorders* 2011; 25:305–20.

Chapter 2

Epidemiology and changing service provision

Key points

- Personality disorder is common and becomes more so as the mental state morbidity of the population examined rises
- Up to 90 per cent of patients in assertive outreach teams may have a personality disorder
- Personality disorder is now recognized as a problem that requires a response from psychiatric services
- Stigma within psychiatric services toward personality disorder remains a challenge to best care

---

2.1 Summary of personality pathology

Although the prevalence of personality pathology is not accurately defined—largely due to classification issues—it is like to fall somewhere in the range of 3–14 per cent of the population. This rate increases dramatically as the psychiatric morbidity of the population examined increases to in excess of 90 per cent of patients in assertive outreach teams. Personality disorder is now well recognized clinically and is no longer a 'diagnosis of exclusion'. The need for an understanding of personality pathology in general mental health services and a place for specialist services involve both clinical and structural input. It is widely recognized that stigma about patients presenting with personality disorder prevents best care and this highlights the needs for ongoing teaching and training.

2.2 The epidemiology of personality disorder in the community

There is disagreement as to the prevalence of personality disorders both in the general population and specialist mental health services. Research suggests that the prevalence of personality disorder varies from as little as 3 per cent to over 90 per cent, depending on the population examined. Inclusion of the important diagnostic classifiers of impairment or distress significantly narrows the prevalence of personality disorder in the community to closer to 10 per cent and 40 per cent in secondary care; however, community samples vary from under 3 per cent to approximately 14 per cent, or one in seven in the general population (Table 2.1). This identifies personality disorder as a major health burden and one of the most common mental health problems presenting to secondary care services, even if it is not always recognized. It

Table 2.1 Study methods and prevalence of personality disorder from recently published epidemiological studies

Author, year (ref.)	Country	Method	Prevalence (%)	Screening instrument
Huang et al., 2009 (6)		Household surveys Multiple imputation used to predict personality disorder scores using a three-part simulation procedure. Rates of personality disorder calculated as means of multiple imputation prevalence estimates (n = 21,162)		33-item screening questions from the International Personality Disorder Examination (IPDE)
	Western Europe (WE)		WE: 2.4	
	Colombia (C)		C: 7.9	
	Lebanon (L)		L: 6.2	
	Mexico (M)		M: 6.1	
	Nigeria (N)		N: 2.7	
	People's Republic of China (PRC)		PRC: 4.1	
	South Africa (SA)		SA: 6.8	
	United States (US)		US: 7.6	
Coid et al., 2006 (3)	England, Wales, Scotland	Survey of a stratified sample of 15,000 households (n = 628)	4.4	Screening questionnaire of SCID–II
Grant et al., 2004 (7)	United States of America	Random sample (National Epidemiologic Survey on Alcohol and Related Conditions) (n = 43,093)	14.8	Alcohol Use Disorder and Associated Disabilities Interview Schedule, DSM-IV Version

Used with kind permission from World Psychiatry. Tyrer, P. et al., Personality disorder: a new global perspective. *World Psychiatry* 9.1 (2010): 56–60.

is therefore likely that clinicians working in general practice will see a personality disordered patient daily and clinicians in a generic psychiatric community mental health team or inpatient setting will be working with multiple patients with personality disorder. Being equipped to understand and manage some of the difficult and challenging issues these patients present is necessary for the clinician. In specialist psychiatric settings, prevalence rates rise dramatically and this almost certainly reflects the potentially enduring and difficult nature of personality problems. It may be that generic community workers become 'burnt out' and refer onwards rather than continue to treat. These are patients who are routinely supported by tertiary services. Geographically diverse studies suggest that personality disorder is not solely a concept in western psychiatry; diagnoses are identified globally.

The variability in prevalence highlights a general problem when understanding personality disorder in both the published literature and clinical practice. Although the variability described can, in part, be explained by the changing population studied, it also reflects the difficulties in making consistent diagnosis. This is a problem reflected in research and clinical work, with a significant disconnect between the two making the easy translation of personality disorder research into clinical practice difficult. It is worth noting that personality disorder is not the only field in mental health to face such difficulties. For example, the prevalence of attention deficit hyperactivity disorder (ADHD) varies widely, with similar problems surrounding its specification, and this disorder is thought to be at the opposite end of the biological spectrum in psychiatry, existing as a largely neurodevelopmental condition.

2.3 The epidemiology of personality disorder in mental state disorders

Studies have also examined rates of personality pathology in the presence of specific mental state disorders. This is clinically relevant as many patients with mental health problems have chronic and enduring illness and may have major personality problems that go undiagnosed for some time. It is also relevant as most referrals to secondary psychiatric services are to assist in the management of mental state disorders that are difficult to treat. Comorbid personality disorder in patients with depression has been most expansively studied. Using strict criteria up to 35 per cent of patients with depression have comorbid personality disorder (more than one in every three depressed patients) in secondary care. Similar figures are commonly found with other comorbid mood problems. The prevalence of PD in anxiety disorder mirrors that of depression and this is perhaps unsurprising considering the overlap between these two mental state disorders. Surprisingly, the prevalence of personality problems in bipolar affective disorder is less well researched; however, figures of close to 30 per cent have been reported. This raises the possibility that underlying factors accounting for much of the difficulties associated with treatment resistance in depression, bipolarity, and anxiety may also be related to personality problems which are poorly recognized and are not managed. Rates of comorbid PD are significantly more variable in psychotic mental disorder ranging from 4.5 per cent to 100 per cent. This variation is in part related to diagnostic issues but it is also related to country of investigation, study type, and instrument used to diagnose personality disorder. Personality can be assessed adequately in the presence of psychosis although the personality profile may vary somewhat from those with a primary affective disorder. In patients with substance use disorders, the prevalence of PD is greater than 50 per cent. In the case of alcohol use disorders, it is not clear which disorder predisposes to the other; however, there is no evidence for an 'alcoholic personality'. In short, it is common for personality dysfunction, and disorder, to be present in many patients who present with a primary mental state disorder, such as depression or schizophrenia, and considering personality pathology specifically remains a necessary, albeit challenging clinical task, as described in Chapter 14.

2.4 **The changing nature of health services towards personality disordered patients**

There is increasing recognition from the providers of public mental services that appropriate funding to resource the management of personality pathology adequately is cost effective. Personality problems have traditionally been considered beyond the remit of both psychiatry and public mental health services, with funding descriptions for services often written up specifically to *exclude* those with personality problems. This approach not only leads to a significant burden of morbidity on those excluded from care but also increases presentations to other parts of the health and justice systems due to problems with behavioural disturbance, often leading to conflict with self (in the form of NSSI) or others (such as verbal or physical violence). The 2003 policy paper published in England, 'Personality Disorder: no longer a diagnosis of exclusion', announced a paradigm shift in the provision of psychiatric care to these patients which has led to steady improvement in services, both generic and specialized, to manage personality problems. Despite this, the attitudes of those working in public mental health services continue to stigmatize patients with personality problems, and there remain issues in terms of the recognition and acceptance of the importance of personality pathology within psychiatry from the perspective of public health. For example, the Royal College of Psychiatrists' anti-stigma campaign did not explore the issue of personality pathology and the public's view of it. Personality problems get short shrift in campaigns in Australasia ('Like minds like mine') and the USA ('What a difference a friend makes'). There are, however, improvements in the ability of public mental health services to manage personality problems if they are identified and this in turn leads to a decrease in the pressures placed on other parts of the social system.

Key references

Newton-Howes, G., Tyrer, P., North, B., Yang, M. The prevalence of personality disorder in schizophrenia and psychotic disorders: systematic review of rates and explanatory modelling. *Psychological Medicine* 2008; 38.8:1075–82.

National Institute for Mental Health for England. *Personality Disorder: no Longer a Diagnosis of Exclusion. Policy Implementation Guidance for the Development of Services for People with Personality Disorder*, Gateway Reference 1055. London: NIMH(E), 2003.

Tyrer, P., Mulder, R., Crawford, M., Newton-Howes, G., Simonsen, E., Ndetei, D., Koldobsky, N., Fossati, A., Mbatia, J. Barrett, B. Personality disorder: a new global perspective. *World Psychiatry* 2010; 9.1: 56–60.

Westen, D. Divergences between clinical and research methods for assessing personality disorders: implications for research and the evolution of axis II. *American Journal of Psychiatry* 1997; 154:895–903.

Chapter 3

Current understanding of personality and its development

Key points

- Western medicine has long recognized that personality is a legitimate area of investigation
- Freud and early analysts laid the foundation for the current predominantly psychotherapeutic approach to personality disorder treatment
- Emerging biological evidence identifies both genetic and neuroanatomical facets to personality traits
- Psychometric testing clusters personality traits into three to seven common groupings

3.1 Summary of understanding personality in medicine

Personality has been recognized by some as a key aspect of medical care since the inception of Western medicine. Consideration of treatment started In the twentieth century with the talking therapies of Freud, and psychotherapy remains the mainstay of treatment today. Building on the psychoanalytic understanding of personality, statistical techniques have been used to cluster personality symptoms into three to seven factors. There is an increasing understanding of the potential biological and neuroanatomical underpinnings personality, and of personality disorders themselves.

3.2 Early development of personality in medicine

The importance of understanding and recognizing the impact a patient's personality has on health has been understood from the earliest days in the development of Western medicine. Hippocrates in the fourth century BCE identified four 'humours' and interpolated these into his theories of health. He described each humour as being related to a bodily fluid and the balance of these fluids essential to a balanced person. In his treatise, *De temperamentis*, he hypothesized about how this balance of hot/cold and wet/dry humours was necessary, the correct amount of blood, black bile, yellow bile, and phlegm, ensuring balance in personal and social life. This concept was further developed by the Roman physician Galen (131–200 CE), who expanded on Hippocrates ideas and sorted four temperaments into categories: sanguine, choleric, melancholic, and phlegmatic. The first of these describes the pleasure-seeking person, extroverted and out-going, as opposed to the choleric temperament of the ambitious leader who is often prepared to go to any lengths in order to achieve his aims. The melancholic personality is not described as depressed, but instead thoughtful and introverted, while the phlegmatic persona describes a relaxed and gentle approach to life. What is immediately obvious from this brief description is the recognition by these early physicians not only of the importance of personality in the presentation of disease but also the fact that personality is ubiquitous and requires consideration as part of medical assessment. In many medical spheres today this interplay between temperament and disease highlights the impact of personality generally. These early writers did not, however, consider personality itself as being a disorder, rather it is the lens through which disease was seen. This concept is re-emerging, in which personality is considered as a diathesis through which disorder may arise, or normal personality facets taken to their extreme describing disorder. Despite this, the clinical utility of the categorical diagnosis remains prominent, and this is reflected in the recent iteration of personality for DSM-5 which retains ten specific personality disorders.

3.3 The psychoanalytic approach to personality

Little work was done on understanding personality further until the emergence of psychoanalysis with the work of Freud in the late nineteenth and early twentieth centuries. A neurologist by training, he initially developed the concept of the unconscious as a driver for mental state disorder (termed 'neurosis') and later developed a sexual theory of psychological development in which various infantile and childhood stages were passed through in order to reach maturity (Table 3.1). This theory is one of the seminal concepts in the development of a contemporary understanding of personality disorder (and its treatment through therapy), however, analysis is used increasingly less frequently in public mental health services. This is partly because it is time-consuming, expensive, and does not fit well with the modern biomedical approach. In the latter years of his career, Freud developed a theory of the psyche as existing in three parts, the ego, id, and super-ego. More complex and coherent than his sexual theory, this schema layered these three parts of the psyche over the notions of conscious, preconscious, and unconscious psychodynamic mechanisms of brain function. Freud posited that most of the psyche was unconscious and a balance between these psychic elements was necessary to develop emotional stability. Although Freud did not specifically describe these in terms of personality structure, his conceptualizations describe the development of normal adult personality, making the assumption that fractures in this development led to mental disorder.

Freud and his immediate successors used these theories to develop 'talk therapy', the term initially used in relation to the treatment of Bertha Pappenheim, better known as Anna O.

Table 3.1 The Freudian stages of personality development according to the 'sexual theory'

Stage Name	Age	Description
Oral Stage	Infancy	Described as the pleasure of breastfeeding
Anal Stage	Toddler	Related to the development of bowel control
Phallic Stage	Childhood	Fixation on parents as sexual objects ('Oedipal complex')
Latent Stage	Adolescence	Reintegration of the trauma of the phallic stage
Genital Stage	Adulthood	Sexual maturity

The goal was to treat neurosis, the early formulation of primarily depressive and anxiety disorders. These 'talk therapies' form the basis for management of personality pathology in current clinical practice, albeit current applications are theoretically and practically divergent from that used by Freud. The utility of psychotherapy is highlighted in most national practice guidelines and reflects the implicit understanding that developing a greater understanding of the self is an essential element of personality management.

3.4 The biological evidence

There is a growing body of literature that is starting to describe the genetic and neurobiological basis of many personality facets. Some research has been conducted which directly examines personality disorders as described using the categorical DSM system, although much focus is on personality traits such as impulsivity as endophenotypes, rather than using a categorical formulation. This is driven by the evidence that points to a trait-based personality structure rather than discrete personality disorders as currently described.

Genetic studies have focused on quantitative and molecular methods to define the genetic basis of personality endophenotypes. Estimates of heritability in personality traits range from 30–60 per cent with multiple unknown genes purported to have small additive effects. It is not clear how directly these studies map onto personality disorder. Studies examining PD as clusters (clusters A, B, and C) have generally taken a dimensional approach that leans towards trait descriptions, even when the term 'personality disorder' is used. Within cluster A personality disorders, schizotypy is most heritable and the conclusions drawn from this suggest schizotypal personality disorder is better considered part of the schizophrenia spectrum, as it is classified using the ICD system, sharing common genetic traits. Other cluster A personality disorders—paranoid and schizoid—have lower if still significant heritability closer to 30 per cent with some evidence for genetic clustering of these traits. The same research group has replicated the methodology to characterize genetic heritability for cluster B and cluster C groupings. In cluster B PD common genetic factors account for 24–48 per cent of the variance in the data (with histrionic PD least genetically influenced and antisocial PD the most) with few shared environmental factors. Interestingly, antisocial personality disorder (ASPD) and borderline personality disorder (BPD) appear to be genetically interlinked. In the cluster C grouping, heritability ranges from 27–35 per cent although in this group, obsessive compulsive personality disorder is genetically distinct, suggesting it is not sensibly grouped with the other cluster C disorders. Factor analysis of clinical assessments would broadly mirror these genetic findings. Molecular genetics, looking for specific candidate genes, has identified a number of possibilities, although this research remains emergent. Candidate genes in schizophrenia coding for dysbindin, D-amino-acid oxidase, and catechol-O-methyltransferase are also found in schizotypy, linking cluster A PD with psychotic mental state disorders. In a similar fashion, the genes coding for proteins found in the serotonin/dopamine/noradrenalin pathways have been implicated in cluster B PDs although most of these studies have not been replicated.

Imaging studies have been used to identify brain structures associated with personality disorder, with borderline and schizotypal personality disorder being the most studied. Many of the imaging findings are from single reports and the findings are appropriately tentative. Frontal structures involved in regulation of impulsivity and emotion are targets for research with reduction in the ventral medial cortex (R) and orbital frontal cortex (L) identified in BPD. Neuroimaging using positron emission tomography (PET) shows reduced metabolism in similar brain areas. In schizotypal personality disorder the findings are mixed, but changes appear to fall on the spectrum between normal and schizophrenia.

3.5 **What can personality instruments tell us?**

In a similar fashion to the development of an increasing biological understanding of personality, the last two decades have seen a proliferation of peer-reviewed scales measuring both normal personality and personality disorder. These have grown out of two distinct line of research: exploration of normal personality and efforts to more accurately identify abnormal personality or personality disorder. The development of instruments that allow grouping of patients is essential to allow for further research; it is difficult to examine an intervention strategy in a group of people with personality pathology if they do not share similar traits! Early researchers identified a small number of general personality traits existing within people which was followed by attempts to measure and cluster these traits accurately and in a reproducible way. Statistical analysis allows for quantification of trait markers and factor analysis simplifies the complex data sets into manageable groups of factors. In practice, this involves asking many people a series of questions (usually 100–300) with this data reduced to between one and seven factors. Test re-test reliability in the questionnaires allows for further refining in order to remove questions that do not discriminate. Although this approach leads to reproducible results and a high degree of internal reliability, validity is open to criticism. The terms used to name each factor are within the researchers' control and indeed the number of factors identified is somewhat arbitrary, particularly if exploratory factor analysis is used. This means many of the tools designed using a factor analytic approach (and this includes most of the current PD questionnaires) identify a variable number of factors and the naming of these factors is widely disparate, even if similar traits are being described. This can diminish the clinical utility of the tools (and the factors themselves). No one tool has emerged as the most clinically relevant or has taken precedence in clinical practice. These tools are more useful in clearly identifying personality facets and allowing research using similar approaches and tools to be compared.

3.6 **Psychometrics and normal personality**

Some of the best-known tools designed to measure normal personality using the factor analytic approach are the scales designed by Paul Costa and Robert McCrae. First published in 1976, Costa and McCrea identified a three-factor structure to personality. This included the extroversion–introversion axis and the anxiety–adjustment axis, both well identified, and a new third factor labelled openness to experience. It was not until 1985 that the five-factor model was published. The two 'new' factors refined the statistical analysis; labelled agreeableness and conscientiousness. Costa and McCrea used the statistical approach of factor analysis to explore both higher-order and lower-order factors in personality questionnaires. The researchers noticed that higher-order factors appeared to group together in a very consistent way. By examining the content of the individual questions, Costa and McCrae identified these five 'core' personality domains, known by the mnemonic OCEAN (Table 3.2). The first factor, described as 'Openness', explains the trait of enjoying or being open to new experiences. This can be in the internal domain (such as fantasies) or in the real world. Conscientiousness describes the personality facets of self-control, diligence, a desire to achieve, and a natural tendency to order. Extroversion is perhaps the oldest recognized personality trait of the modern era, first noted by Eysenck in 1947 (also using factor analysis). Costa and McCrae identify this as the sensation-seeking trait, being outwardly focused, assertive, and overflowing with energy. Agreeableness is the trait of being trusting, listening, and tending to believe the explanation as it stands in a straightforward manner. Finally, Neuroticism is described as an inbuilt sense of anxiety with a tendency to depressive rumination and hostility. Many of the normal personality questionnaires in existence today follow a similar pattern as the original, albeit with different monikers (Table 3.2). It is interesting to note that the model developed using factor analysis is

Table 3.2 The domains of the five-factor model of Costa and McCrea for normal personality traits: similarities with other modern models

Author				
Costa and McCrae^	Conscientious	Extroversion	Agreeable	Neuroticism
Hippocrates	Sanguine	Phlegmatic*	Choleric*	Melancholic
Cattell (1957)		Extroversion		
Norman (1963)	Conscientious	Surgency	Agreeable	Neuroticism
Tyrer and Alexander (1979)	Anankastic	Schizoid*	Sociopathic*	Passive-dependent
Mulder & Joyce (1997)	Anankastic	Asocial*	Antisocial*	Asthenic
Clark. (1996)	Impulsivity*	detachment	callousness	dependency
Asendorpf et al., (2001)	Undercontrolled*			Overcontrolled
DSM-IV		Cluster A*	Cluster B*	Cluster C
DSM-5		Cluster A*	Cluster B*	Cluster C

- ^= Openness is omitted as it maps poorly to other personality traits listed by others.
- * = These traits lie at the opposite end of the spectrum described by Costa and McCrae (I.e. they reflect the antithesis of the described trait).
- # = Cattel is included here as this work was a fundamental building-block in modern personality delineation. He described sixteen personality factors.

Source: data from Tyrer, P., Coombs, N., Ibrahimi, F., Mathilakath, A., Bajaj, P., Ranger, M., Rao, B., Din, R. Critical developments in the assessment of personality disorder, *British Journal of Psychiatry*, Volume 190, Supplement 48, pp. s51–s59, Copyright © 2007.

similar to that observed by Hippocrates and Galen over 2,000 years ago. This is in stark contrast to psychodynamic theories developed early in the twentieth century. What is also obvious is that we all have, to some degree, each of these character traits and 'too much' of any of them could potentially cause conflicts with others or internal dysregulation, the hallmarks of personality disorder as it is defined in both DSM-5 and ICD-11. The 'big five' tool is, however, designed to identify personality characteristics in the *normal* population and is not focused on personality disorder, despite the two being interwoven. This raises the question of how normal personality and personality disorder are related.

Key references

Bouchard, Jr. T. J., Loehlin, J. C. Genes, evolution, and personality. *Behavior genetics* 2001; 31(3):243–73.

Costa Jr, P.T., McCrae, R.R. (1976). Age differences in personality structure: A cluster analytic approach. *Journal of Gerontology* 1976; 31(5):564–70.

Freud, S. The ego and the id. Standard Edition 1923, 1–66.

Grey, S. Evidence and Narrative in Contemporary Psychiatry. *Journal of the American Academy of Psychoanalysis and Dynamic Psychiatry* 2009; 37(3):415–20.

Mulder, R. T., Newton-Howes, G., Crawford, M. J., Tyrer, P. The central domains of personality pathology in psychiatric patients. *Journal of Personality Disorders* 2011; 25(3):364–77.

Torgersen, S., Kringlen, E., Cramer, V. Dimensional representations of DSM-IV cluster B personality disorders in a population-based sample of Norwegian twins: a multivariate study. *Psychological Medicine* 2008; 38(11):1617–25.

Tyrer, P. Personality diatheses: a superior explanation than disorder. *Psychological Medicine* 2007; 37(11):1521–6.

Chapter 4

Normal personality and personality disorder

Key points

- Personality disorder is separate from mental state disorder, and identifies people whose personality causes them harm in their interaction with others and society
- Personality disorder changes over time: most personality pathology ameliorates over time although schizoid type traits may become more pronounced
- Although a dimension approach to personality is probably closer to the biological construct, a categorical approach has been retained by DSM-5 to maximize clinical utility. A dimensional descriptive approach is included for further research
- Collateral history is an important part of assessment
- Severity may be of greater clinical relevance than the specific personality disorder for management purposes

4.1 Summary of normal and abnormal personality

Personality disorder is generally considered to comprise personality problems that cause significant personal distress or social impairment. Difficulties in cognition, emotional control, interpersonal functioning, and impulse control are core features. These features are pervasive but changeable over time. Many personality traits that cause difficulty ameliorate over time, most notably impulsivity and antisocial traits. Conversely, schizoid traits tend to harden. Although debate remains as to whether a categorical or dimensional approach to diagnosis is most appropriate, the categorical approach is used in DSM-5 and ICD-10. Understanding severity allows for clinical decision-making as to what management may be most appropriate and its timing.

4.2 What makes personality 'disordered'?

Debate remains as to whether 'personality disorder' as a concept differs in some way from normal personality; are the two in fact one and the same? Identifying a categorical disorder suggests a difference from extremes of normal personality leading to interpersonal distress and conflict with society. The term 'personality disorder' appears at first unusual, possibly pejorative, as it presupposes there is something about a person's personality, identifiable in a reproducible way, that is sufficiently damaged to be labelled disordered. The concept of reproducibility underlies structured interviews and this is different from the unstructured approach taken in clinical practice. The difficulties with clinical accuracy using an unstructured approach may explain some of the reluctance to use the term in a clinical setting. Nonetheless, it is increasingly obvious that there are people for whom the concept of self is sufficiently disturbed to cause major, potentially life-threatening, changes in behaviour, gross disturbance in thoughts, and affective instability in the absence of mental state disorder. It is this basic tenet—the personal and societal disability caused by the conflict between personality structure and society—that defines personality disorder. This depends both on the trait characteristics of the individual as well as the societal mores and values within which a person lives. For patients with such problems, identifying the personality disturbance may bring a sense of order and the possibility of help. Although research into personality most strongly supports a dimensional approach to diagnosis, a categorical approach is considered to provide greater utility clinically in identifying patients who are likely to respond to treatment. Bearing this tension in mind, understanding the characteristics that identify personality disorder helps in the consideration of management strategies.

4.3 The general characteristics of personality disorder

The defining characteristic of personality disorder is a disturbance in an understanding of self and others that is sufficient to cause major problems in everyday functioning for the person concerned. The disturbance in a notion of self is widely recognized and variously described using difference critical lenses, depending on the perspective of the author. The psychodynamic approach labels difficulties with understanding self as 'identity disturbance', whereas a cognitive behavioural model may see this as disrupted understanding of core belief formation. From a clinical perspective, the patient is likely to give a history that shows an extreme lack of ability to consider the world away from his or her direct experiences and he or she may understand his or her own experience in a rigid way. There is often little sense of self containment, with poorly developed boundaries between self and others. Accompanying this is a diffuse sense of self direction and a lack of autonomy. This, perhaps unsurprisingly, leads to major difficulties in attaining happiness or feeling fulfilled. This is very different from the presentations usually found in mental state disorder (Table 4.1). In terms of interpersonal interactions, the primary

Table 4.1 The differences between personality disorder and mental state disorders

	View of self	Interpersonal management
Personality disorder	Often fractured Little clear notion of self Over-reliance on feedback from others Few or no internal checks and balances	No concept of others experiences Socially gauche Relationship related to power Little reciprocity in relationship
Depression	Negative self-worth Poor self esteem Little concept of future	Sees others as judging Avoids socialization Tires easily in interactions
Anxiety disorder (generalised anxiety, phobias)	Increased self-monitoring Vigilant to internal cues Expectation of disastrous outcomes	Struggles with interpersonal contact Increases self-monitoring Assumes negative views from others
Mania	Overtly positive Unrealistic self-expectation Self as 'perfect'	Little regard for others Others as subservient Lacks empathy
Eating Disorder	Perfectionistic Body focused Overly rigid	Variable
Autism	No clear view of self	Usually disturbed by seeing people as objects

problem lies in developing a rich internal mental world from which representations of others are positively formed. This leads to an over-reliance on an egotistic perception of the world and desire to avoid harm at almost all cost. Due to the difficulties in seeing the world from another's perspective, relationships tend to be based on the emotional ability to receive comfort (or pain) with little reciprocity. This leads to an overvalued perception of rejection that can lead to significant dysregulation of behaviour. For these problems to be considered an element of personality disorder, both problems with self and interpersonal relationships need to be present, and there needs to be a clear history of problems throughout a significant proportion of adult life.

4.4 The longitudinal course of personality pathology

One of the difficulties in the diagnosis of personality disorder is the variance between the diagnostic classification systems currently in use and the growing body of literature with respect to abnormal personality characteristics over time. Both the DSM and ICD state that personality problems are recognizable from early adulthood and present in a continuous fashion. There is now evidence to suggest that the dimensional traits of normal personality may be stable over time but the impairments in interpersonal functioning and behaviour, related to disorder, are not. It is increasingly clear that not all personality pathology develops linearly and evidence suggests that fulfilling the requirements for temporal stability for categorical diagnoses, even in the most studied and clinically diagnosed personality disorder, BPD, is fraught. Narcissistic, histrionic, and self-destructive personality traits tend to ameliorate over time. Conversely the rigid, perfectionistic, introspective personality traits tend to become more apparent as time progresses. As the population studied becomes older, the overall rates of personality pathology therefore decline, with a changing pattern of presentation. Histrionic, narcissistic, borderline, and antisocial personality disorders tend to become less apparent, with an increase in other PD presentations. In practice many patients may appear to 'grow out of' a personality disorder such as borderline PD, and others may 'develop' new schizoid personality disorders later in life. None of these personality trait changes occur in a linear way meaning that over the course of months or years, patients may come close to fulfilling the diagnostic criteria but they may not either have or develop any categorical personality disorders. It is also clear patients who do not fulfil the diagnostic criteria for a particular category may have multiple minor problems and fulfil the criteria for personality disorder 'Not Otherwise Specified' (PD-NOS). These patients are less well-studied as to their longitudinal course, although they have similar psychosocial morbidity as other personality disordered patients. The clinical picture is not, therefore, as straightforward as the diagnostic rubric suggests.

4.5 The categorical versus the dimensional approach

What is clear is the ability exists to identify patients without mental state disorder who have clinically meaningful disturbances in personality functioning, but often not in a way that maps easily onto the categorical diagnostic criteria traditionally used. Although different from the development of normal personality characterization, the concept of personality disorder identifies behavioural and interpersonal disturbances that can be present to varying degrees. Personality facets are naturally multi-dimensional, with different degrees of impact depending on the person and there environment. Personality disorder can be defined as the overlaid disturbances that can result from a combination of these traits, environmental stressors, and early experience. Despite the greater scientific precision of dimensional approaches, there is challenge in using a dimensional approach in the binary decision algorithm of to treat or not to treat. This is true of many areas of medicine, such as cardiovascular disease (e.g. blood pressure) and infectious diseases (e.g. temperature), where categorical cut-offs provide significant clinical utility. These measures are, however, more simplistic than trait assessment.

One of the major advances in the understanding of personality disorder was the development of the categorically distinct personality disorder diagnoses, placed on axis II in DSM-III. Not only did this spur on research, it endeavoured to provide discrete entities for clinicians to use diagnostically. Unfortunately these categories have proved far from discrete with PD-NOS, the most commonly use diagnosis in research, and multiple personality disorder diagnoses often present in the same individual. This has led to confusion around the clinical utility of a categorical approach and around the diagnosis itself. Despite this, a categorical approach may be able to identify those patients who are most significantly impaired by their personality profile and this may have the advantage of continuity from a research and clinical perspective, rather than the adoption of a purely dimensional approach. Most experts agree that the current categorical lexicon falls far short of its lofty ambition, however, there is little agreement as to what should replace it. This emphasizes the need for clinical utility, while removal of the 'NOS' classifier and axis II reinforces to clinicians and researchers the need to be deliberate in the use of categories and consider dimensional description when clinical personality problems exist but when they do not fulfil the categorical diagnostic rubric (Table 4.1). The exception to this 'rule' is borderline personality disorder where the diagnosis has become increasingly clinically identifiable. Associated with this, a number of evidence-based treatments have emerged (see Chapters 11 and 12).

4.6 **The importance of information gathering**

What is necessary to be able to identify confidently the presence of personality disorder in routine clinical practice? This is an area often relatively poorly taught in clinical training and may explain some of the difficulty in accurate diagnosis. It is not, however, difficult and it simply requires an altered emphasis in the standard psychiatric interview. It is almost always necessary to interview a patient on multiple occasions to identify personality disorder and to confirm the enduring nature of the problems associated with it. The exception to this is where there is a clearly documented prior diagnosis, with a history that describes the basic problems of personality pathology (Box 4.1). History should involve an assessment of the patient's early childhood, focusing on experiences of interpersonal trauma, separation, and adult attachment figures. A pattern of intra- and interpersonal problems often exists before early adulthood

---

Box 4.1 Essential elements of personality disorder assessment

- Clear history of negative impact on development from adverse life events
- History of difficulties in understanding of self from early adulthood
- Problems in relationship in multiple domains, e.g. family, school, peers, work colleagues, and intimate relationships
- Social functioning at the extreme end of normal or frankly unusual in multiple domains, e.g. no friends, constant conflict with others, rejection of family, inability to maintain any employment
- Behaviours that cause direct (e.g. deliberate self-harm, suicide attempts, dangerous drug consumption) and indirect (e.g. avoidance of others, uncontrolled aggression, rigid relationships with social bodies) harm to self
- An enduring pattern of behaviour

and this is usually highlighted in problems with schooling and the transition from family to peer affiliation. Understanding the interpersonal history, focusing on conflict and tension, provides important information as to how a person functions in their most important relationships, and questions that ask the patient for their views and reflection of these allows for a clear conceptualization of the patient's ability to be empathetic and self-reflective; characteristics commonly impaired in personality disorder. A medical history focusing on risks to self, including various types of non-suicidal self-injury (NSSI) and the personal response to self-harm is essential to understand a patient's strategies for managing distress, and inform the development of a risk-management plan. If hazardous use of alcohol or illicit drugs is present, understanding the antecedents to use aids in differentiating between behaviours associated with the compulsive nature of addiction and personality disorder (use to manage emotions, numb psychic pain, etc.) is extremely important. As the history gathered from patients with personality disorder may be scanty on first presentation, repeat interviews are almost always necessary and collateral information is important. Reviewing prior medical and psychiatric notes clarifies the type of presentations and the dangerousness associated with them. Communication with the GP may also provide valuable insight into the patient's presentations over years from an objective perspective. Collateral history from family provides context as they may have a much greater understanding of patterns of behaviour, particularly interpersonally, than the patient themselves. Finally, information from a partner (if present) may assist in identifying discrepancies in the patient's perspective of his or her day-to-day functioning and may offer an objective assessment. If the patient refuses to allow contact with others, engagement and working with the patient to help him or her understand the need for this can be helpful.

4.7 Severity and its clinical impact

What has also become clinically more relevant is the increasing recognition of the impact of severity in association with personality pathology. If present it is often the degree to which personal abnormalities play out behaviourally that causes the most distress, and this is directly related to the severity of the disorder present. Although this does not make the use of categorical descriptors invalid, it highlights the clinical need to identify severity and triage management in response to this. Severity can been measured in many ways including number of symptoms present, number of personality disorders present, direct counts from personality disorder questionnaires, and general functionality measures such as the global assessment of functioning (GAF). Severity is often related to the number of contacts made with healthcare services in all areas (including the emergency room, general practice, and psychiatric services), and the severity of internalizing behaviours leads to self-harm. As severity increases, so does the urgency for appropriate management strategies. It is likely that behavioural disturbance associated with severity requires the most urgent clinical attention and longer-term psychotherapy requires a reduction in severe behavioural disturbance for maximum effectiveness.

Key references

Bernstein D. P., Iscan, C., Maser, J. Opinions of Personality Disorder Experts Regarding the DSM-IV Personality Disorders Classification System. *Journal of Personality Disorders* 2007; 21(5):536–51.

Clark, L. A. Stability and Change in Personality Pathology: Revelations of Three Longitudinal Studies. *Journal of Personality Disorders* 2005; 19 (October):524–32.

Cohen, J., Nestadt, G., Samuels, J., Romanoski, A., McHugh, P., Rabins, P. Personality Disorder in later life: a community study. *British Journal of Psychiatry* 1994; 165:493–9.

Krueger, R. F., et al. Deriving an empirical structure of personality pathology for DSM-5. *Journal of Personality Disorders* 2011; 25(2):170–91.

Skodol, A., Gunderson, J., Shea, T., McGlashan, T., Morley, L., Sanislow, C., Bender, D., Grilo, C., Zanarini, M., Yen, S., Pagano, M., Stout, R. The Collaborative Longitudinal Personality Disorders Study (Clps): Overview and Implications. *Journal of Personality Disorders* 2005; 19(5), October:487–504.

Yang, M., Coid, J., Tyrer, P. Personality pathology recorded by severity: national survey. *British Journal of Psychiatry* 2010; 197:193–9.

Zanarini, M., Frankenberg, F., Hennen, J., Silk K. The longitudinal course of borderline personality psycho-pathology: 6 year follow up of the psychopathology of borderline personality disorder. *American Journal of Psychiatry* 2003; 160:274–83.

Chapter 5

Cluster A personality disorder

> **Key points**
>
> - Cluster A personality disorders lead to socially isolated patients who do not routinely seek treatment
> - Although not psychotic, symptoms may significantly restrict the lives of patients with cluster A personality pathology
> - Risk is less of a factor than with other personality pathology
> - Schizotypal personality disorder is related to schizophrenia

5.1 Summary of cluster A personality disorder

Cluster A personality disorder includes schizoid, schizotypal, and paranoid personality disorders. These disorders share some clinical and management features with the psychotic disorders and schizotypal is most closely aligned with this mental state disorder grouping. Often patients with cluster A PDs minimize or have little concern about their difficulties; however, appropriate management may significantly improve their overall wellbeing. It is usually most appropriate to manage patients with cluster A PDs in the community.

Schizotypal PD is classified in the schizophrenia spectrum in the ICD-10, and this reflects the neurobiological data finding similarities between schizotypy and schizophrenia. Although many people with cluster A PDs may not fit well in society, they do not generally see themselves as having much of a problem and rarely present themselves to services for help. More frequently it is parents or other family members who become increasingly concerned about their loved ones and the drift away from normal development. From a clinical perspective, this leads to a gradual reduction in social contact and increasing amounts of time in one's own company. Associated with this the patient may become more socially gauche or dismissive of others. This can lead to problems in maintaining normal relationships with old friends and family, and it considerably restricts work opportunities.

5.2 Epidemiology

As with many personality prevalence studies, clarity about the burden of these personality disorders in the community is challenging. Early studies identified a prevalence of 1.6 per cent in Western community samples; however, this increases significantly in high-risk groups, such as those with close family members with psychotic mental disorder. Longitudinal studies suggest a chronic, albeit mixed, pattern of development commonly associated with this group and the age of the patient group needs to be noted. As age increases, the prevalence of some odd traits increases, however the group as a whole shows a moderate amelioration over time. An additional challenge in interpreting these studies is the relative lack of contact with services notable in patients with these personality types, and the subsequent potential for under-reporting.

5.3 **The clinical presentation**

Clinically patients with 'odd' personality disorder may not be willing presenters to primary or psychiatric services. Although they see little problem with their chosen lifestyle the conflict with others, who are often concerned about them, may lead to such presentation. It would not be uncommon for this to occur after repeated 'did not attend' appointments. Occasionally the degree of concern from others leads to an assessment under mental health legislation, a situation that adds challenge to the clinical interview in patients who are often cold, aloof, and lack empathy. Such patients may not only be relatively disinterested in review but also somewhat suspicious and detached from the interview process. It is likely that they do not understand the causes of concern noted by others and may well not endeavour to explain or justify their behaviour. A notable lack of rapport is obvious early in the interview process and these patients may engender a feeling similar to patients with psychotic disorders, but without the obvious positive symptoms. The interview is likely to progress slowly with little information offered except by direct questioning and little recognition of this as potentially causing difficulty. An example of this is given in the case of Mr GL. The pattern of interpersonal interaction that emerges is either of long-standing mistrust of others or an increasing disinterest in the lives of others. Both lead to gradual social withdrawal or a drift away from social contact that offers the patient little, or they may find actively threatening. This drift leads to a restriction in the patient's ability to enjoy the company of others, and they may struggle to identify joy in their lives. There may be conflict with those whom they feel are prying unjustifiably into their lives, however it is unlikely that this will be delusional. One common example is the demand for interview itself. Work is uncommon for these clients and if found is usually in an isolated job where little contact with the outside world is required. The older the patient, the more likely these patterns will be rigid and increasingly less amenable to challenge at interview, particularly if the patient has schizoid traits. From a psychosocial perspective, these clients are unlikely to be particularly concerned about their physical appearance or the environment within which they live, and this can lead to concerns about the ability to maintain basic care of self. They may be unkempt and malodorous at interview without this being noticeable to them. The primary differences between the specific cluster A diagnoses are described in Table 5.1.

5.4 **Risk assessment**

Little in the way of risk to self and others is usually identified, with a lack of personal hygiene and care in one's appearance the most notable problems. It may be that these problems reach such a degree that neighbours or councils may become concerned about the patient's accommodation and hygiene. In some settings, however, patients with the odd personality disorders may be at particular risk where their aloof style may conflict with others in their environment. The problems with interpersonal interactions may only become obvious when someone is promoted from an isolated job to one where they are obliged to interact and manage people. Although these patients may be very good at working alone, moving into interactive workplace environments are likely to be both threatening and overwhelming, potentially triggering a referral for psychological review.

Table 5.1 Primary features of the cluster A personality disorders: schizoid, paranoid, and schizotypal		
Paranoid	Schizoid	Schizotypal
Highly suspicious of others	Socially isolated but does not want relationships	Magical thinking
Untrusting of sharing personal information	Little sexual interest	Ideas of reference
Does not trust others generally	Enjoys solitary activities	Unusual thinking and speech
Looks for the negative message in communications	Few hobbies or joys	Paranoia
Bears grudges	Indifferent to praise	Restricted affect
Is vexatious in regards to perceived threats	Emotionally cold	Unusual behaviours
Doubts partner	Few or no close friends	Few or no close friends

5.5 Sources of information

As with any psychiatric assessment, considering collateral sources of information is important in ensuring a comprehensive assessment is completed. For patients with odd personality disorders, the completion of formal psychometric tests can be useful because these individuals present a myriad of assessment difficulties at interview. There are many scales that can highlight paranoid or schizoid traits and this taxon (schizotypy) has been clarified over the last three decades. Although this measure (and others) should not be considered diagnostic, it may help in clarifying the diagnosis when the clinical picture is not clear. It is worth noting that there is debate about the use of tools to identify the odd personality disorders, and some have argued that, for example, schizoid personality disorder is best conceptualized by avoidant and/or schizotypal personality traits. Collateral information from family and (if available) friends is also of benefit as it provides another picture of interpersonal problems, longitudinal decline, and a description of the person's capacity to interact in the world. GP and other formal medical files are often not a good source of information as patients with odd personality disorders usually do not see problems in themselves and are unlikely to present regularly to these services.

5.6 Setting of care

When thinking about initial steps in treatment, the best setting to consider is in the community, often in the patient's own home. There is likely to be little benefit from hospital admission which in any case may lead to either a significant increase in distrust in the purpose of the assessment or stress at being surrounded by many other (unwell) people. Some explanation of the diagnostic formulation and the reasons for treatment at home may help to alleviate the concerns of parents or others in the initial stages. Any intervention is best thought of as an 'n 1 trial' in discussions with the patient, thinking about what changes may occur and the timeframe for these. The patient may be able to reflect on the potential for improvement and consent to an intervention on these grounds as Mr GL did (see the case vignette Mr GL). Weighing up the patient's capacity to consent and engage in treatment versus the natural inclination to withdraw is important in ensuring that any management strategy is implemented in an ethically sound way while acknowledging the problems leading to presentation. Clearly, enlisting the support of family and others is helpful in this regard. Regular DNAs should be expected initially.

Case vignette—Mr GL

Mr GL, a 27-year-old man, came to the attention of psychiatric services after a referral by his employment assistance program (EAP). He had been to see his EAP as he had recently received a promotion at work and had been struggling to cope since this time. The counsellor in this program was worried Mr GL may be developing schizophrenia, hence the referral. Mr GL arrived at his second appointment having missed his first, and he felt the need for psychiatric review was unnecessary. He did not think he was 'crazy', and had checked on the Internet and did not think any of the symptoms described for a psychotic mental disorder fitted him. He denied having any difficulties in his early childhood, raised within a nuclear family. He agreed he was less sporty than his two siblings but denied any particular problems at school, and had successfully completed his exams. He described some bullying by fellow pupils during this time and became a 'loner', feeling he was also bullied by his teachers. His parents did not listen to his concerns and he stopped discussing his worries with anyone. After leaving school, he moved away from home and found employment on a waste-disposal truck, having found a university course too challenging. He enjoyed this work, starting at 3 o'clock in the morning and finishing at 10 o'clock so that he could spend the rest of the day on the Internet. He struggled to identify joys outside work. He agreed that from time to time he felt his 'truckies' would pick on him and he had little contact with family after a falling out with his father. Mr GL explained that his father had called him a 'loser' because of his employment and felt that his son was not pushing himself hard enough. He reported that occasionally, he believed that others were monitoring his Internet activities and was concerned that this would limit his time on the computer. He had no further explanation for this but agreed it troubled him. Approximately three months earlier, he had received a promotion to a role managing the truck at work. This meant being responsible for coordinating the personnel each day, finding cover for sick or absent personnel, and attending a weekly meeting at head office. He agreed that this was stressful but he knew he had the 'brains' to do the job. He wondered if he had been given the promotion so that if he did not succeed, the company could fire him.

A diagnosis of probable paranoid personality disorder was made and treatment initiated with a low-dose antipsychotic. Its off-licence use and the reasoning for the diagnosis and treatment choice explained to Mr GL. It was agreed a three-month 'trial' would take place to assess for any change due to the medication. After three months the patient was reviewed. He had no problems with his medication and reported no side effects. He agreed his job was more manageable and no longer believed the promotion had been made in order to eventually fire him from the company. He had been able to ask to be excused from the weekly management meetings via his EAP and had used the extra remuneration to upgrade his computer security. He asked to continue the medication as, on balance, he felt better using it despite not acknowledging there had been any problem prior to starting treatment.

Key references

Lenzenweger, M., Lane, M., Loranger, A., Kessler, R. DSM-IV personality disorders in the National Co morbidity Survey Replication. *Biological Psychiatry* 2007 15 September;62(6): 553–64.

Triebwasser, J., Chemerinski, E., Roussos, P., Siever, L. J. Schizoid Personality Disorder. *Journal of Personality Disorders* 2012; 26(6):919–26.

Tyrer, P., Mitchard, S., Methuen, C., Ranger, M. Treatment Rejecting and Treatment Seeking Personality Disorders: Type R and Type S. *Journal of Personality Disorders* 2003; 17(3):263–8.

Chapter 6

Cluster B personality disorder

Key points

- Narcissistic and histrionic personality traits are common in society although the prevalence of disorder is poorly identified.
- Disorder occurs when these traits lead to personal and/or social morbidity
- Managing patient contact often requires a team approach with clear communication essential

---

6.1 Summary of cluster B personality disorder

These personality types are dramatic, flamboyant, and are often the centre of attention. The need for this focus usually has detrimental consequences for them and may lead to repeated presentations to psychiatric services. Information from family and friends can help to highlight the social problems caused. Risk assessment needs to consider the possibility of positively reinforcing behaviours if overt attention is paid to harmful acts.

Of all the personality trait groupings, the dramatic cluster is perhaps the most controversial as to what features are core to its presentation and how these are represented over time. Despite this, it is the dramatic presentation (including borderline personality disorder, which will be discussed in the next chapter) that comes to the attention of medical services most frequently and is often correlated with social morbidity and mental state disorder. Juxtaposing this, both histrionic and narcissistic traits tend to lead to minimal contact with health services. These traits in people tend to lead to exaggerated positive beliefs about self in relation to others, rather than internal problems or behaviours that cause social problems. The literature is unclear as to exactly how this group is best considered with considerable overlap and sub-grouping in factor analytic studies and systematic reviews. Due to the weight of evidence in borderline personality disorder, this diagnosis is discussed separately in the next chapter and the present chapter focuses on histrionic and narcissistic personality pathology (Table 6.1). Antisocial personality disorder is not considered in this handbook, and both psychiatric and social problems caused by this disorder tend to be managed by judicial or forensic services.

6.2 Epidemiology

Clarifying the prevalence of dramatic personality presentations is difficult owing to the similarity of these disorders to traits found in the general population and the relative reluctance to acknowledge or seek support for interpersonal and social problems. The large-scale National Epidemiologic Survey on Alcohol and Related Conditions in the USA investigated the rates of narcissistic personality disorder and estimated a population prevalence of 6.2 per cent.

Importantly this study also noted the significant overlap with other mental health problems and social difficulties. The initial wave of this prevalence study found 1.8 per cent of the population fulfilling the criteria for histrionic personality disorder, giving a combined estimate of 8 per cent of the population with these two disorders. It is worth noting, however, that the prevalence of these personality subtypes in the general population is variable, with international studies indicating the histrionic, borderline, and narcissistic personality disorders may be closer to 1.5 per cent when considered as a unitary construct, and as low as 2 per cent for the cluster as a whole in the USA. This suggests some of the expression of these traits may be dependent on the society in which people live and the methodology used for data collection. This gives clinicians a glimpse of the impact of social and methodological factors influencing our understanding of personality pathology. For disorders such as these it is likely that prevalence rates will continue to change as social mores evolve and methods of diagnosis become increasingly robust.

6.3 Clinical presentation

Patients with dramatic personality disorders need to be the centre of attention, admired and praised by others, as is highlighted by Ms RR. They expect to be surrounded by sycophants and often have a powerful and negative reaction when this does not occur. Related to this, patients with dramatic personality structures tend to act in a way that requires them to be noticed and if this does not occur in day-to-day life, they may create situations in which this happens, even if this is ultimately to their detriment. In these situations their personality become clinically relevant, with 'acting out' occurring at home, the workplace, and with friends to such a degree that it interferes with normal social functioning. The interpersonal problems that may arise include inappropriate sexual advances or the consistent demand for attention that is not warranted by knowledge, understanding, or position. Unsurprisingly this causes conflict and may lead to psychiatric intervention. Occasionally the responses of others to such behaviour are poorly considered, or may not be thought important at all. At interview these patients are likely to impress upon the clinician their relative 'specialness', and act and talk in such a way as to make this clear. Indeed, they may be quite likeable, even charming on first impression, but as the interview progresses a sense of emptiness or arrogance may emerge. They are likely to play down any event that may potentially cause them to be seen in a negative light, and this may make it difficult to be clear as to the extent of problems they have had in multiple domains. Open-ended questions are likely to be answered increasingly vaguely and closed questions should clarify areas of ambiguity, although the process may well be somewhat laborious. By the conclusion of the interview, both parties are likely to be somewhat frustrated, the patient with the psychiatrist's fixation on problems, and the doctor with the client's reluctance to be open about the difficulties in his or her life and what role he or she plays in these.

6.4 Risk assessment

Patients with dramatic presentations present two distinct types of risk, to themselves and to the treating team. Initially these patients may come into contact with services due to acting-out behaviour that may place them in harm's way. If this behaviour engenders a powerful positive reinforcement (e.g. they become the sole focus of attention), there is an increased risk of repetition of similar behaviours in order to engender a similar response. Being mindful of this potential for positively reinforcing self-destructive behaviours allows the clinician to consider the short-term benefits and risks and weigh these against the longer-term pros and cons of any action. These behaviours may also lead to conflict with others and this may place relationships with family, friends, and work colleagues in jeopardy. Managing this risk is similar to the approach taken with borderline personality disorder patients. Individuals with narcissistic problems are also at higher risk of alcohol and drug dependence and the difficulties associated with these problems, and this risk needs to be assessed also. The other risk these patients pose is to the clinicians assessing and managing them. These patients need to be special or the centre of attention and are likely to respond negatively to feeling like one of many. This may lead to reactions to reinforce their 'special-ness' if they feel under-appreciated, such as complaints to registering boards or advocacy services. This is likely to consume significant proportions of a health practitioner's time and is therefore a way for the patient to meet their internal drives. If the complaint is of a personal nature (such as a complaint of inappropriate behaviour) this can have a lasting impact. To manage such risks, clinicians should be aware of this potential and monitor for it. Team working becomes increasingly important, and the clinician should bear in mind the opportunity for both close team communication and seeing patients in pairs. Clear docu-mentation of interactions ensures a contemporaneous record of events should disputes arise in the future and will allow the entire treatment team to remain up-to-date with the progress of interventions.

6.5 Sources of information

Unlike the odd personality disorders, patients with flamboyant personality pathology are likely be more than happy for collateral information about themselves to be collected. There are likely to be many contacts with their primary health care provider with an unusual array of problems and possibly a history of complaints when these are not investigated promptly and fully. They may have many primary care physicians who have struggled to satisfy their demands. Family members are likely to note a consistent pattern of conflict revolving around the need to be the centre of attention, particularly in inappropriate situations such as another family mem-ber's birthday. This may reach the point where there is little family contact as there is a sense that any family event is likely to be disrupted by the patient's mores. Work experience is likely to show the need for promotion and recognition, potentially into roles the patient is unable to fulfil. Failure to be promoted or recognized can lead to extreme distress or arrogant denial of problems, and this may lead to difficulties in maintaining employment.

6.6 Setting of care

It is likely that these patients will not engage in further care if they can avoid it, and using the assessment sessions to formulate the diagnosis and provide feedback is helpful. Ongoing management, if the patient is willing for this to occur, is best undertaken on an outpatient basis. A clear team structure prevents multiplication of work, splitting of the team itself, and minimizes the risks that are associated with these personality traits. Regular assessment pro-vides for continuity and modification of any treatment strategies. Hospital admission may act to reinforce behaviours that have made a person the centre of attention. Angry denial of concerns, disengagement and conflict with services at future contact points are all possible other consequences. Consideration of long- and short-term contingencies is necessary and clear boundaries, even if this causes an initial escalation in dangerous behaviour, may provide for long-term benefits. The notion of self-responsibility is often therapeutically helpful. Reviews should not be undertaken in a way that differs from standard clinical practice and this should be reflected in any care plan. A 'supportive approach' may not be beneficial and indeed may increase the prevalence of disruptive core personality traits.

Table 6.1 Similarities in histrionic and narcissistic personality disorder

Histrionic personality disorder	Narcissistic personality disorder
Needs to be the centre of attention	Grandiose sense of self-importance Requires admiration
Inappropriately sexually seductive	
Shallow and shifting emotions	
Excessively impressionistic speech	
Theatrical	Fantasies of success and beauty
Suggestible	Lacks empathy
Considers relationships as overly intimate	Exploits relationships
	Considers self to be 'special'
	Has a sense of entitlement
	Envious of others
	Arrogant and haughty behaviours

Case vignette—Ms RR

Ms RR was referred to psychiatric services for an assessment of her mental state by a private psychologist. He had been reviewing Ms RR following the breakdown of her marriage, despite recommending to her that she see a specialist marriage councillor. She was unwilling to do this as she needed someone 'more skilled', by her own account. Ms RR explained that her relationship had ended due to the intolerable behaviour of her husband who would pry on her in the house and inhibit her actions. Eventually this had become too much, leading to the separation that had not gone smoothly as, according to Ms RR's account, her ex-partner refused to be reasonable in continuing to support her financially after dividing the assets. She explained she needed to travel and her clothing was more expensive than his and he needed to acknowledge this. She felt her husband simply did not understand this requirement, which existed because she expected to become famous via a blog or journal, and she felt she deserved to be supported until such time as this recognition commenced. She denied depressive, anxious, or psychotic phenomena, other than her unique capacity for understanding people. There was no family history of mental disorder although Ms RR understood her parents were not her intellectual equals and this caused some stress. Although denying any problems with alcohol or drugs, Ms RR stated on careful questioning she would drink between a half and a full bottle of wine, five to six nights per week, but she stated this was not of concern because she did not drink in the same way as her ex-partner. She described an idealized childhood and claimed to be the 'perfect' wife and stay-at-home mother to an eight-year-old child, neither being adequately recognized. Although initially reluctant to attend the interview, Ms RR agreed that it was helpful to see such a skilled physician and asked for a further appointment, in a private capacity.

A tentative diagnosis of narcissistic personality disorder was made and confirmed over several interviews (in a public setting). The lack of effective pharmacotherapy was discussed and the potential for therapy to help Ms RR understand interpersonal problems better was recommended. Ms RR agreed to this but abruptly ended the sessions when the diagnosis of narcissistic personality disorder was discussed in more detail, and this was followed by her registering a complaint to two health professional registering bodies.

Key references

Mulder, R. T., Newton-Howes, G., Crawford, M. J., Tyrer, P. J. The Central Domains of Personality Pathology in Psychiatric Patients. *Journal of Personality Disorders* 2011; 25(3):364–77.

Stinson, F. S., Dawson, D. A., Goldstein, R. B., Chou, P., Huang, B., Smith, S. M., Ruan, J. W., Pulay, A. J., Saha, T. D., Pickering, R. P., Grant, B. F. Prevalence, Correlates, Disability, and Co morbidity of DSM-IV Narcissistic Personality Disorder: Results from the Wave 2 National Epidemiologic Survey on Alcohol and Related Conditions. *Journal of Clinical Psychiatry* 2008 July; 69(7): 1033–45.

Chapter 7

Cluster C personality disorder

Key points

- Anxious, dependant, and avoidant personality disorders cause significant morbidity and present as 'low-grade' anxiety and mood disorders with a chronic course
- Patients internalize symptoms but would generally like to be more comfortable in the presence of others
- Standard psychiatric risk assessment and management is usually sufficient

7.1 Summary of cluster C personality disorder

Cluster C personality disorders represent the fearful group, with features leading to internalization of problems and difficulties in managing interpersonal relationships. Although these problems usually diminish with age, it can be difficult to differentiate the normal anxieties of transitional stages in late adolescence from early disorder. Obsessive–compulsive personality disorder is categorized with this group, although much of the clinical presentation and biological evidence suggests they may be better classified on their own. Risks are usually able to be managed in the community.

Juxtaposing the presentation of the dramatic and odd personality disorders, individuals in the fearful or anxious group display the core characteristic of being overly concerned at how they exist in the world and what the world's view of them is. These problems are largely internalizing although the impact of the environment on functioning cannot be overlooked. This anxiety is usually sufficient to prevent these patients from effectively interacting in the workplace, managing family relationships, and finding fulfilment in the activities of day-to-day life. These problems are often related to the process of development in the emerging adult personality and care is needed in considering fearful personality traits in young adults, particularly if there is disruption in the family home. Whereas dramatic or odd personality problems may track their way back into adolescence (or even childhood), it is developmentally normal to be somewhat anxious during the transition from childhood to adulthood when one is finding one's place in the world, and this differentiates this cluster of personality traits from the others. The stability of personality traits improves throughout the life course, with most stability in the 50–70-years-old range.

7.2 **Epidemiology**

Anxious/avoidant, dependant, and anankastic personality disorders[1] are stable in the community, with the first two of low prevalence although OCPD is reported as the commonest PD in some community samples. It is probable that the true rates approximate 2, 0.5, and 8 per cent respectively. There is also a significant overlap with mental state disorders that are anxiety-driven including depression, generalized anxiety disorder, phobic disorders, and PTSD. This can add challenges in differentiating personality pathology, a temporally stable trait-based problem in multiple domains, from these state-based disorders if a cross-sectional approach is use in research in the clinical setting.

7.3 **Clinical presentation**

Fearful patients are often insightful into the restrictions bought about by their temperament and are minded to do something about this. They are quite likely to self-present although they may struggle to attend due to fear of rejection or minimization of the problems perceived by others. Rapport is likely to be good and patients can usually provide a comprehensive history. It is likely the patient will emphasize difficulties as a child and at school in forming and maintaining friendships, and this may be at the extreme end of the spectrum. Their attachment style as a child is likely to be disorganized, with elements of anxious–avoidant behaviour in their history, although these are not defining characteristics (Table 7.1). As patients describe their interpersonal relationships in life, these become increasingly restricted in number of contacts and by depth of relationship. A common theme relates to fear of rejection leading to avoidance of interpersonal connection or increasingly dysfunctional attempts to maintain them. Mr LK's case highlights many of these points, some of which may appear within the range of normal if not considered as a whole and within the patient's social context. The overly rigid style of OCPD tends to lead to increasing conflict with others, and it also progressively limits contact. A consequence of this is evidence of efforts to hold on to relationships already formed. From a pragmatic perspective these problems can be expressed as difficulties in making decisions, struggling to engage in interpersonal debate, and an inability to cope interpersonally. Unlike cluster A PDs, these patients want to maintain their relationships and feel the loss of them keenly. These problems make functioning in a group setting difficult and undertaking basic tasks such as managing the home can become insurmountable. Over time, this style of interaction can cause increasing difficulties for loved ones and children, and it may be these concerns that prompt the decision to seek medical attention. Unlike anxiety and depressive mental state disorders, these symptoms are chronic, 'low-grade', but functionally highly impairing. In fact the dysfunction may be greater than that caused by depressive disorder alone. It is the loss of functioning that usually prompts referral to psychiatric services, a process often occurring over many years. Longitudinally, these problems may worsen over time and behavioural patterns become rigid.

7.4 **Risk assessment**

This category of patients does not generally present with major risks to self or others that can be differentiated on the basis of personality pathology alone. This does not mean they carry no risk, rather that general psychiatric screening for suicidality and risk to others is generally sufficient. Developing a generic management plan as part of general psychiatric care would generally be expected to provide for appropriate management strategies.

1 There is also some argument as to whether obsessive–compulsive traits are best thought of as similar to other fearful trait disorders or whether they perhaps fulfil their own distinct group. This remains unclear, but for the purposes of clinical utility these problems are discussed in this chapter.

Table 7.1 DSM-5 characteristics of cluster C personality disorders

Avoidant	Dependent	Obsessive–compulsive
Isolates from other due to fear of criticism	Struggles with decision-making	Constantly sets rules and boundaries and rigidly adheres to them
Expects to be disliked	Avoids responsibility	Attention to detail prevents completing jobs
Remains fearful even in close relationships	Won't disagree with others	Overly focused on productivity
Expects rejection in social situations	Activities are rarely solitary	Morally inflexible
Feels inadequate	Needs constant reassurance from others	Tends to hoard objects
Sees self without strengths	Often feels helpless when alone	Is poor at delegating
Doesn't take personal risks	Cannot tolerate being with-out a partner	Spends little and anxious about money
	Fears potential abandonment	Is stubborn

7.5 Sources of information

Patients themselves may be a rich resource, usually providing a clear picture of longstanding problems with avoidance and anxiety. Primary care physician notes will often have entries associated with contact, often for a presumed anxiety disorder, and trials of antidepressant/anxiolytic medications are not uncommon. The literature is conflicted as to the responsiveness of these disorders to pharmacotherapy and therefore although the history itself is useful, response to treatment provides little discriminate utility in separating mental state disorder from personality pathology. The family will be able to provide an account of an increasingly restricted life, with fewer and fewer social contact that causes the patient distress (unlike schizoid patients).

7.6 Setting of care

Like the odd and dramatic groups, initial treatment is best trialled at home although there may be a place for group work if this is unsuccessful. Bearing in mind the likely long history and comorbidities (with addictions, anxiety and depression), placement within a therapeutic community setting (if available) may in fact provide for greater change related to the structured environment. This form of learning by experience may be of value but is poorly evidenced for this group. A combination of structured community care and routine liaison with other involved service providers is likely to be most beneficial in order to provide appropriate intervention without the patient becoming too dependent on the service or services provided.

Case vignette—Mr LK

Mr LK, a 34-year-old gentleman, was referred for psychiatric assessment by his GP who explained he had made a diagnosis of obsessive–compulsive disorder but Mr LK appeared treatment-resistant. The GP wondered if a second opinion and cognitive behaviour therapy (CBT) might be appropriate. Mr LK described his problems as a difficulty in discarding items from his home and increasing stressors at work managing a team involved in software design. Mr LK agreed he had always enjoyed collecting objects, although what these were tended to change (currently it was old transistors) and were generally of little financial worth as he was concerned about his financial position; this was despite his having no outstanding debts other than a small mortgage. Mr LK explained he was single partly by his own choice as he did not like the 'loose ways' of current society and others appeared to have difficulty understanding his outlook. Mr LK denied depressive, anxiety, and psychotic symptoms. Specifically Mr LK denied intrusive thoughts; instead, he insisted he had clarity as to how he saw the world and was frustrated by the opinions of others. This was now becoming a major problem at work were he had put three of his nine staff under close management to ensure that they were productive despite no history of prior problems with them and no complaints. Mr LK agreed some saw this as micromanagement. His managers were now asking him to explain this and the paradoxical reduction in customer satisfaction associated with it. Mr LK could not understand how his careful attention to the work being done could possibly be a bad thing. Mr LK described a normal childhood as a single child of a 'neurotic' mother and absent father. He had few friends, due to the foolishness of others. He had intimate relationships in his life but these ultimately led to separation, and he found this upsetting.

A diagnosis of OCPD was made and the reasons for this made clear to the GP, particularly the absence of ego-dystonic intrusive thoughts and compulsive behaviours. Psychotherapy was commenced via a third-wave CBT approach, acceptance and commitment therapy, and psycho-education, rather than exposure and response prevention. After six months Mr LK was able to return to his old role at work, had ordered his objects at home, and had a clearer understanding of his personality style. He was exploring options to return to dating and described his outcome from therapy positively.

Key references

Crawford, T. N., Cohen, P., Midlarsky, E., Brook, J. S. Internalizing Symptoms in Adolescents: Gender Differences in Vulnerability to Parental Distress and Discord. *Journal of Research on Adolescence* 2001; 11:95–118.

McGlashan, T. H., Grilo, C. M., Skodol, A. E., Gunderson, J. G., Shea, M. T., Morey, L. C., Zanarini, M. C., Stout, R. L. The Collaborative Longitudinal Personality Disorders Study: baseline Axis I/II and II/II diagnostic co-occurrence. *Acta Psychiatrica Scandinavica* 2000; 102:256–64.

Skodol, A. E., Gunderson, J. G., McGlashan, T. H., Dyck, I. R., Stout, R. L., Bender, D. S., Grilo, C. M., Shea, M. T., Zanarini, M. C., Morey, L. C., Sanislow, C. A., Oldham, J. M. Functional Impairment in Patients with Schizotypal, Borderline, Avoidant, or Obsessive-Compulsive Personality Disorder. *American Journal of Psychiatry* 2002; 159:276–83.

Tyrer, P., Rutter, D. The Value of Therapeutic Communities in the Treatment of Personality Disorder: A Suitable Place for Treatment? *Journal of Psychiatric Practice* July 2003; 9(4):291–302.

Chapter 8

Borderline personality disorder

Key points

- BPD is the most studied personality disorder and has features of both personality pathology and mental state disorder
- It is common, can be related to serious NSSI, and requires appropriate assessment and management
- Understanding the difficulties with engagement for these patients prevents inappropriately early discharge to primary care
- Risk assessment can be challenging with short-term and long-term risk management often leading to different conclusions about management. Prolonged hospital-based care may lead to worsening NSSI
- Specialist management is usually warranted

8.1 Summary of borderline personality disorder

Borderline personality disorder (BPD) has been researched more than other personality disorders and often presents to medical and psychiatric services secondary to self-harm. These patients are treatment-seeking, unhappy with their own emotional dysregulation, and have difficulties in coping interpersonally. Dramatic self-harm is distressing for family and emotionally difficult for healthcare staff. Managing risk in this group is of particular importance. Balancing the need to ensure short-term safety against the importance of avoiding positively reinforcing NSSI is difficult and can lead to division within treating teams. Much has been achieved in developing psychotherapeutic treatments for BPD and these treatments have proved to be effective.

Of all the personality disorder diagnoses, BPD is the best recognized, researched, and most common in terms of those patients brought to the attention of general psychiatric services. Despite this, there are questions as to whether BPD is in fact a personality disorder or whether it ought more appropriately to be considered in the mood disorder spectrum. Early in the understanding of BPD, Arkisal famously described borderline personality disorder as an 'adjective in search of a noun', that noun being depression. This is not surprising, bearing in mind the dramatic presentations often associated with this diagnosis and the projection of emotional instability often felt by medical, nursing, and other clinical staff. Patients with BPD often seek treatment then reject what is offered, blaming clinicians for the patient's inability to cope and his or her self-destructive behaviours. Difficulties with managing emotion, termed 'emotional dysregulation', and non-suicidal self-injury associated with BPD are often difficult for staff, families, and patients themselves to deal with. This can leave staff confused, angry, and worried about patient safety and their own professional reputations. Families reflect their loved one's distress, angry at the lack of 'cure', and potentially feel guilty about their own lack of capacity to cope. Patients struggle to cope themselves, unhappy about their lack of internal emotional resources, scared by the overwhelming negative affect they often feel, and upset by the significant self-harming they resort to in order to cope with emotional pain. This volatile mixture of vulnerability and rejection is often one of the most difficult for clinicians to manage, needing clear team structures in place to identify the diagnosis in patients and to develop robust management plans. Although the last part of this handbook is aimed at the treatment of personality disorders in general, due to the nature of the evidence, most guidance presented is based on the management of BPD.

8.2 **Epidemiology**

The prevalence of BPD is well researched and reported in multiple countries and across many samples. Due to the significant use of healthcare services by this group of people, understanding prevalence is important. In community samples, rates of BPD have been reported ranging from 0.7 per cent to 5.9 per cent. As clinical samples with increasing social morbidity and psychopathology are surveyed, prevalence continues to climb, reaching in excess of 90 per cent in assertive community outreach teams. What is obvious from these figures is the significant burden BPD has placed on the healthcare sector and the likelihood that clinicians will see patients with BPD in the course of usual psychiatric, medical, or primary clinical care is high. Evidence also reflects clinical practice insofar as BPD is a diagnosis whose prevalence is affected by age. Over the course of six years, three-quarters of all patients with a diagnosis of BPD will attain remission with low recurrence, making it a diagnosis more prevalent prior to middle age.

8.3 **The clinical presentation**

The clinical presentation of borderline personality disorder is diverse (as are the formal diagnostic criteria for all personality disorders). In DSM 5, five or more of nine criteria are needed for diagnosis. This means there are 256 different ways to meet the criteria for BPD using this nosology. Two patients diagnosed with BPD could potentially share a single clinical characteristic. Having said this, there is a common clinical presentation, as described in the case vignette (Ms RT). This involves elements of help-seeking and rejection, NSSI, dysregulated interpersonal relationships (including those with clinical staff), and difficulties identifying and regulating emotion. Although BPD is more clinically common in the younger age group and in women, this is not solely the case. Patients often self-present to medical staff following an episode of NSSI and are subsequently transferred to psychiatric services for assessment and ongoing management. Non-suicidal self-injurious behaviour, although common, is not a necessary requirement to the clinical presentation and this is often a habituated behaviour designed to displace emotional distress into physical pain. It is also common for patients to reject initial offers of help, or to place the assessing clinician in a position whereby they feel responsible for the patient's actions, particularly risky actions, albeit they are helpless to act. This can lead to direct abdications of responsibility from patient to doctor, for example by the implementation of mental health legislation by way of committing the patient. This intervention, although potentially well-reasoned in the short term, can worsen the long-term outcome by teaching the patient that he or she need not learn to manage his or her own emotional distress as this can (and will) be done by someone else. As assessment continues the clinician is likely to recognize that the patient views the clinician and other members of the assessing team in a highly dichotomous way—some all good, other all bad. This is a reflection of the difficulties patients with BPD have in recognizing within themselves the positive and negative nature of many emotional reactions. It is not uncommon for there to be sporadic routine attendance intermingled with acute presentations, and this is likely a reflection of the shifting emotional sands on which the patient walks on a day-by-day basis.

8.4 **Risk assessment**

The assessment of risk in borderline patients often causes anxiety in family and clinicians, and this anxiety potentially serves the purpose of reducing the anxiety the patient feels him or herself. Family and others generally feel the need for high levels of acute care, concerned that any non-suicidal self-injury portends more serious attempts. There is a greater risk of completed suicide in those who have self-harmed than the general population, and higher rates of completed suicide in BPD, so these concerns are not unfounded. Paradoxically, over-zealous detention under mental health legislation, or admission to an acute psychiatric inpatient bed may reinforce NSSI behaviour by positively reinforcing the need of the patient to share the anxiety he or she feels, thereby increasing the likelihood of further episodes of NSSI. Being aware of this, clinicians may develop a management plan in conjunction with the patient that states this risk explicitly, with a clear focus on self-responsibility for behaviour. Such a plan highlights the normal patterns of emotional dyscontrol and its behavioural consequences, and aims to minimize any positive reward from such behaviour. Alternative strategies to NSSI are written into the plan and developed over time with the patient. Longer-term therapy aims to increase self-control and responsibility, reducing the overall number of NSSI events. Assessment is essential at presentation, and indicators of divergent behaviour in respect of NSSI are warnings of new or highly stressful real-world pressures. At these times, more acutely focused care such as brief hospital admission may be necessary. Recognizing family concern, acknowledging it, and working closely with the family provides a more complete picture of behavioural and emotional disturbance and permits the family (if present) to become part of the overall support team. This also enables the family to avoid becoming emotionally responsible for the behaviour of their loved one. Taking a history from supportive people maximizes the likelihood of accurate assessment. Understanding the nature of the NSSI and the surrounding events enables a clinician to judge if a given episode of self-harm mirrors previous attempts and assess the purpose of such attempts. Discussing the patient's intention (e.g. release of tension, express distress, control emotion, to die) and being aware of the medical risks of any self-harm are also important in being able to assess the probability of immediate repetition. Negotiating with the family, bearing in mind that if a patient returns home the response to any repeated self-harm will initially come from the carers, not medical staff, and ensuring that this support team are aware of such risks and have a plan to manage them reduces anxiety and improves the long-term outcomes. It is also important to bear in mind the stage of the disorder. Patients with well-established BPD are often adept at self-harming, they know how it helps them, and may have established patterns of behaviour that require long-term psychotherapy to manage. For patients with an emergent personality disorder it is likely the clinical picture will be significantly less clear, although a well thought-through assessment can prevent any reinforcing decisions being made by the medical team.

8.5 **Sources of Information**

For patients with BPD there are likely to be many sources of potential information that can be usefully accessed. If possible, parents and other family members will be able to elaborate on the patient's personal history and points of inconsistency can provide insights into the patient's mental state. Family are likely to have a clear understanding of the emotional strain associated with interactions with the patient and the anxieties that emerge because of it. Friends may be able to provide a differing opinion, particularly related to current attachments, and the patient's capacity to manage emotional separation. It is not uncommon for an associate to attend an assessment interview in routine care and for them to have had the experience of being called on to act as 'rescuer' at times of crisis. Review of social media also has the potential to help to give a rounded picture. Many people have a presence on Twitter, Facebook and other social media and the information presented may give a unique insight into the patient's daily life. This is particularly the case with younger patients (Gen-y or 'net-genners'), whose webpages can offer insight into the patient's state of mind and capacity to interact with others outside the clinic. Medical notes, emergency room encounters, and details from primary care appointments will be able to clarify how often the patient seeks help and the degree of dangerousness associated with self-harming behaviours. Finally, liaising with colleagues who know the patient may provide pertinent information as regards previous successful strategies for managing distress and potentially difficult triggers.

8.6 Setting of care

Deciding on the best place to provide care for patients with BPD is, like a great deal of the management of these patients, a potential source of both conflict and anxiety. Where management occurs depends somewhat on the presentation of each patient; however, as a general principle care is best delivered where the patient lives as this is where the environmental stressors that need to be managed exist. The exception to this is where these stressors are judged to be too great, and in these circumstances a brief period of respite (at a friend's, respite facility, or hospital) may be clinically appropriate. The level of respite care relates to the degree of dangerousness with which the patient and situation are judged to present. From a practical perspective, this means the patient is likely to remain at home with a package of care provided by a community mental health or specialist personality disorder service. Although this may cause concerns around the possibilities of further NSSI, prolonged hospital admission does not appear to ameliorate this risk and in some patients, the positive reinforcement associated with hospitalization may act to reinforce dangerous behaviours. Individual plans may involve routine, structured time for patients in a respite facility, recognizing the difficulties for both patients and families that is innate in a community-based approach (particularly initially).

The potential negative consequences of hospital-based care need to be considered at each assessment or crisis as admission may cause an escalation in self-harming behaviour as a means of managing distress. This is accomplished by handing over responsibility for safety to an inpatient team. In some areas there are specialist therapeutic communities designed to provide longer-term inpatient care for patients with personality disorders and people with complex mental health problems that almost always have comorbid personality disorder. These facilities are not acute psychiatric units and they have a community ethos with clients working individually and as a group to manage themselves and the community. This 'learning by doing' approach is anecdotally useful for BPD patients, although it is increasingly scarce due to the high costs associated with its provision.

Case vignette—Ms RT

Ms RT presented to psychiatric crisis services following an overdose of 16 grams of paracetamol leading to emergency room admission. At 27 years old, this was her first presentation to psychiatric services and although reluctant to engage with them, she stated she had taken the overdose after a breakup with her boyfriend. Her mother had come to visit as arranged, found her daughter on the floor with the empty packets of paracetamol in the bin, and had therefore called an ambulance. Ms RT admitted this was not the first overdose she had taken and explained that it was a useful way for her to 'be calm' when she felt out of control. She had initially experimented with the idea when she was 16 after watching a YouTube clip. She did not know how often she took overdoses but guessed it was as often as once a month, generally associated with drinking alcohol. She denied a desire to die. She agreed that self-harming usually occurred after conflict with a friend or partner. She denied feeling depressed or anxious on general questioning. She denied manic or psychotic symptoms but did state she would often feel numb and sometimes felt as if she was watching herself do things without being in control of them. Ms RT described a difficult relationship with her mother, who brought her up after her father left the family home. She recalled her mother frequently fighting with boyfriends but refused to discuss her childhood in any greater detail. She denied problems at school, being academically bright and having a variety of friends and boyfriends, the latter whom she described as 'useless'. Throughout her early adult life, Ms RT worked in office jobs and on two occasions had been dismissed after romantic relationships at work, once with her line manager. She lived alone in rented accommodation and had 'just broken up'. She described herself as hopeless and 'a bad person' and could not describe her feelings in greater detail. Immediately prior to the overdose she said she knew she would be alone forever and could not bear that thought. Ms RT was receptive to the idea of further contact and the interview concluded with Ms RT thanking the team for the review and expressing confidence in them to 'fix me'.

Ms RT presents with classic features of borderline personality disorder with symptoms from late adolescence despite her first presentation to psychiatric services occurring at age 27. These include recurrent self-harming, a diffuse sense of self, and related difficulties in her interpersonal relationships. Her self-harm appears driven by a need to avoid abandonment and to elicit a positive and caring response from others. It continues despite evidence that it does not achieve this aim. She describes using NSSI as a means for managing emotional distress. The descriptions of dissociation and difficulties with feeling empty, signals mood instability and a poor understanding of self. Other mental state disorders need to be ruled out (or identified comorbidly), as do physical problems. It is rarely appropriate to definitively identify personality disorder on a single assessment in the emergency room, however, there are sufficient indicators to recommend a further community assessment and psycho-education around risk management with the patient and any support she may have in the community. Education for her mother may also be beneficial in providing short-term support for Ms RT. Collecting collateral history from RT's mother (and ideally the boyfriend), GP records, and emergency department notes will identify other undisclosed hospital visits. A review of her Facebook page may clarify and support her account of events, helping to guide appropriate management.

Key references

Akiskal, H. S., Chen, S. E., Davis, G. C., Puzantian, V. R., Kashgarian, M., Bolinger, J. M. Borderline: An adjective in search of a noun. *Journal of Clinical Psychiatry* February 1975; 46(2):41–8.

American Psychiatrists Association. Practice guidelines for the treatment of patients with borderline personality disorder, *American Journal of Psychiatry* 2001; 158:295–302.

Grant, B., Chou, S., Goldstein, R., Huang, B., Stinson, F. R., Saha, T. D., Smith, S. M., Dawson, D. A., Pulay, A. J., Pickering, R. P., Ruan, W., J. Prevalence, Correlates, Disability, and Comorbidity of DSM-IV Borderline Personality Disorder: Results from the Wave 2 National Epidemiologic Survey on Alcohol and Related Conditions. *Journal of Clinical Psychiatry* 2008 April; 69(4): 533–45.

Zannerini, M. C., Frankenberg, Hennen J., Silk, K. The longitudinal course of borderline psychopathology: 6 year follow up of the phenomenology of borderline personality disorder. *American Journal of Psychiatry* 2003; 160:274–83.

Chapter 9

General principles of personality disorder management

Key points

- Assessment of personality disorder differs from a standard psychiatric assessment in focus rather than requiring a new skill set
- Being aware of personal responses to crises allows for clear decision making
- Considering short- and long-term benefits is important.
- Patients should, whenever possible, remain responsible for their actions
- Risk assessment is dynamic and ideally involves the wider team, patient, and their support network

9.1 Summary of the general principles of personality disorder management

Personality disorder management requires a comprehensive approach as do all mental disorders, although a focus on antecedent events and risk has increased priority in this instance. Diagnostic assessment usually takes longer, but correct diagnosis is very important. Being aware of potentially difficult personal responses to personality disordered patients allows for reflective practice and minimizes burnout. Usually a team approach is best with clearly defined roles and responsibilities.

9.2 Is the management of personality disorder any different from mental state disorders?

As the assessment, recognition, and management of personality pathology increasingly becomes part of standard community and inpatient mental healthcare, the need to understand the general principles of personality disorder management becomes equally important. Essentially the management of personality disorder is no different from managing a mental state disorder, but there is a change of emphasis in response to the unique challenges associated with this group of patients. Although the present and following chapters largely relate to borderline personality disorder, the principles outlined particularly in this chapter apply to all personality pathology. The management focus on borderline personality disorder reflects the state of the current literature rather than any particular emphasis on this being a more important or disabling disorder than any other.

As with any referral to services, ensuring an adequate assessment in order to be clear about diagnosis is the first and most important step. If personality disorder is suspected, this process usually occurs over the course of many interviews, unlike mental state disorder which can be diagnosed relatively quickly. Trait classifiers are part of normal personality functioning and their use can sometimes be misleading if clinical personality disorder is present. DSM-5 now recognizes the importance of personality disorder that does not fit into a diagnosed category but continues to cause significant problems. Rather than use the NOS classifier, DSM-5 now includes the diagnoses of 'other specified personality disorder' or 'unspecified personality disorder'. A dimensional construct in part three of DSM-5, with specifiers, allows patients with personality disorder to be appropriately diagnosed within the major domains of difficulty and severity thereof. This is potentially an improvement in both clinical utility of the PD diagnosis and aligns more closely to the scientific evidence that the majority of personality disorders are more accurately considered in terms of dimensions rather than as categories. Using a psychometric assessment tool can confirm the diagnosis if doubt exists but this is not generally used in clinical care. Once diagnosis is clear, building a therapeutic team to address the various biopsychosocial issues present is helpful. This often means involving a psychiatrist who can consider diagnostic, risk, and general management issues, a skilled therapist (or therapy team) ideally using an evidence-based approach for personality pathology (see Chapter 10), and case manager to undertake routine community assessments, liaise with the family, assist with developing a risk plan, and who can provide overall coordination with community services. Review in the larger multi-disciplinary team provides for support from the whole service to the managing team and ensures everyone is involved in building a management plan. Issues here to emphasize if personality pathology is identified include: managing engagement, initiating family involvement in care, clear risk-management planning, and contingency planning. As various parts of a service will be involved in the movement from management to recovery (e.g. a crisis team, the emergency room, the inpatient team), clear communication is essential because personality disordered patients are more likely to divide teams as a reflection of their internal difficulties. This has the potential to create gaps between services, the treating team, and the wider MDT. These splits are thought to reflect the patients' internal dichotomies, they act to reflect the dysregulation within the patient. The need for review and discharge planning also provides points of stress, with the potential for issues of abandonment, perfectionism; reward-seeking, and reassurance making this process difficult. Clear, structured planning at an early stage is important in order to manage this transition well.

9.3 **The general principles of individual patient interaction**

Although a large part of the management of patients with personality disorder follows similar pathways as management of those in psychiatric care, when considering the interaction with a patient and with particular regard to the internal difficulties the patient is likely to be battling, a variety of factors need to be borne in mind. First, and possibly most importantly, giving the patient as much control over the process of recovery as possible is important. This ranges from how and when they engage in treatment, to what (if any) medication they take and how they are reviewed. This makes clear that the patient's task is to move towards improved psychological health and ensures that they are taking responsibility for their actions, finding ways to manage both behaviourally and cognitively. The therapy team's task is to guide this process, provide specific skills and insights (for example, through therapy), liaise with others to provide education and understanding, and ensure the progress to recovery occurs in as safe a manner as possible. This is somewhat at odds with the current biomedical model used in psychiatry which can disempower the patient and lead to a myriad of ongoing problems. Second, there needs to be recognition that much of the evidence for the management of personality disorder is weak and occasionally divergent.

Interventions therefore need to be carefully designed as '$n = 1$' trials. Patients need to be clear prior to starting treatment about what the potential benefits are, but they should also understand that the possibility of treatment failure exists. This both increases engagement and mitigates against a catastrophic response if the treatment fails. The timescale within which to expect benefit is also important to clarify prior to the initiation of treatment. Third, risk-management planning requires careful consideration of the balance between short-term risks and long-term risks associated with an intervention. For example, allowing a patient to hold all their medication may increase the risk of overdose but it empowers him or her to be responsible for managing his or her mood and impulsivity using appropriate pharmacotherapy. This risk assessment is dynamic and requires regular and frequent evaluation in light of the patient's course. Risk management also includes a collaborative (if possible) approach to developing a plan to deal with crises, ensuring the rationale and actions consider both the long- and short-term pros and cons of any acute intervention. Finally, sufficient clinical time (both with the patient and after seeing them) is required to ensure that a strong plan is developed under the auspices of good team working. An example of a risk-management pro forma is provided in Figure 9.1.

Every patient with a personality disorder will, in some way, resonate with our own experience, and ensuring that there is team support for the decisions made allows for objectivity and clarity in future planning. This can be difficult in high-risk cases, and seeking external expert review is often of significant benefit. Case consultation can provide another opinion as to what drives psychopathology and whether the management plan may benefit from alteration. It is also just good clinical practice.

9.4 Personal responses to personality disordered patients

Perhaps more than other group of patients, those with personality disorder can leave clinicians feeling overwhelmed, and this can led to negative attitudes in those clinicians who attempt to help this patient group in their recovery. It is easy to feel exhausted by the day's end. This is probably due to the emotional difficulties associated with this client group. The chronic stress of potential suicide is also greater and direct threats about this made by patients in the earshot of their clinicians are not uncommon ('you can't help me and you're the expert; I may as well just go and kill myself now because you can't help me!'). Recognizing these stresses lets clinicians reflect and manage them. As there is a wide range of personality profiles, it is difficult to predict in what way personal responses are likely to cloud clinical thinking. Confusion can be minimized by close team working and appropriate supervision or peer review. Some evidence-based treatments recognize this and they incorporate specific times for therapists to meet together in order to discuss patient progress (for example, mentalization-based therapy and dialectical behavioural therapy). The presentations most likely to arouse a strong emotional response will come from patients diagnosed with a cluster B disorder, including antisocial and borderline disorders. Patients with these disorders often appeal to the clinician's professional responsibility to help as well as the clinician's own narcissistic traits and may try to make the clinician feel special, and particularly responsible for them. This can lead to situations where the clinician, for example, feels a need to admit a distressed patient to hospital in order to fulfil their 'unique' role despite a careful plan which they have developed with the patient not to do so. Being alert to possible personal responses helps the clinician to ensure appropriate decision pathways are followed. The team approach also protects against the possibility of crossing professional–personal boundaries.

9.5 **Risk planning**

Risk planning plays a key role in the management of personality disordered patients as many of these patients pose a dynamic risk to themselves and others. As discussed earlier, it is the repeated presentations to the emergency room, primary care, and other general medical settings that often causes so much distress to family and stress on medical staff. All self-harm is potentially life threatening and needs to be taken seriously; dying is one outcome from self-harming behaviours (Box 9.1). It is important to remember that for a patient's family and friends, the experience of NSSI in a loved one is uncommon, scary, and portends more serious future behaviours. This 'baseline experience' is often quite different to that of clinical staff who can be frustrated and angry at what can be seen as waste of their time and energy. If not recognized and managed, this tension can escalate potential conflicts between patients, families and medical carers that may increase the risk of further self-harming. An example of a joint crisis plan is provided in Figure 9.1. It recognizes potential triggers and situations that are likely to increase emotional dysfunction or arousal. The common pattern(s) of behaviour in response to this are identified and more functional management strategies outlined. Crisis measures to be taken when all other strategies fail are noted including the need for respite and the level this respite might take. As patients progress through therapy, this may include 24–48 hour hospital admission at the patient's request. From the patient's perspective, recognizing this comprises taking responsibility for unmanageable thoughts of self-harm and suicide and initiating appropriate action to protect him or herself and his or her loved ones. As no two patients are the same, each plan requires unique input and consideration.

9.6 **Managing self-harm**

With respect to managing the risks associated with NSSI, the first step is taking a thorough history. Elements of the history to focus on include: understanding the antecedents to the behaviour (self-harm), the intended purpose of the act and immediate response, how the self-harm came to medical attention, and the potential lethality. This allows the clinician to assess the likelihood of very serious (or fatal) outcomes from further self-harm episodes more accurately, and this guides management. Recognizing patterns assists in this judgement. For most patients whose self-harm is related to personality pathology (often in the dramatic group), it is essential

Box 9.1 Indicators of increased lethality from NSSI	
Background factors:	Childhood physical abuse
	Childhood sexual abuse
	Male gender
Current factors:	Multiple social problems (women only)
	Alcohol dependence
	Drug dependence
	Comorbid psychiatric disorder
	Difficulties with housing
	Eating disorder (women only)
	> 1 cluster B personality disorder

Figure 9.1 Pro-forma risk plan for the personality disordered patient. This is one element of the overall management plan.

Health care informtiaon

Patient Details (name, address, ph):

Health care details (Psychiatrist name and team, GP details, other inputs)

Family contacts in a crisis:

Diagnoses(medical and psychiatric):

Medication (psychiatric and non-psychiatric):

History of self-harming(when, where, what, how, who aware):
1.
2.
3.

Unhelpful actions in a crisis in the past:

Helpful actions in a crisis:

Reminders for me in a crisis:

Triggers for a crisis often include:

Unhelpful behaviours in response to this can be:

Helpful alternatives to try include:
1.
2.
3.

Responses from the psychiatric service/active service/emergency room that I would like are:

Review Date

Staff signature and date   Patient signature and date to allow them to maintain as much control over and responsibility for their actions as possible, and to supersede this only if the risk is judged to be life threatening. Taking an overly cautious short-term approach can increase the risk of repeated self-harm and a poorer long term prognosis. Casting a careful eye towards long-term risk is perhaps the most important judgement a clinician can make in managing self-harm in personality disordered patients. As discussed, ensuring clear communication with family, GP, the emergency team, and the various elements of the psychiatric service is also vital to enable everyone to understand and participate in the risk-management plan. This prevents a split in the team and provides a clear and consistent message to the patient.

9.7 Providing seamless care

Identifying the members of the team, their roles in care and managing emergencies provides for best care. Usually the role of the psychiatrist is to ensure correct diagnosis, to coordinate the care, to discuss issues and concerns with the family, and to consider pharmacotherapy (see Chapter 10). A psychologist is usually important, playing a role in developing a therapeutic alliance and delivering evidence-based psychological treatment (see Chapter 11). Many therapies are delivered as a team and there are likely to be other therapists involved here. A case manager in the general team allows for day-to-day assessment, acts as a point of contact for the patient, and is key to implementation of the crisis plan should it be needed, enabling the therapy team to concentrate on recovery rather than managing crises. The blurring of therapy and crisis management is a common pitfall. Regular discussion with, and inclusion of, the crisis response teams is also important. These are likely to include the psychiatric crisis team, psychiatric ward, accident and emergency, and primary care. Contact between all enables a clear and consistent message to be given to the patient, the coordination reflecting the goal of increased intra-psychic connection. Review of the plan by a specialist personality disorder service can offer a useful second opinion and is beneficial from a clinical governance perspective. Wider MDT input is also important in order to ensure the whole team is aware of the major issues related to each patient. Last, treatment takes time, and ensuring any changes to the team occur in a careful fashion with appropriate handover prevents patient deterioration relating to feelings of abandonment or rejection.

Chapter 10

Pharmacotherapy for personality disorder

> **Key points**
>
> - Pharmacotherapy is generally not the first-line treatment for personality disorder
> - Many patients with personality disorder are on three or more medications without any evidence of effectiveness. Monotherapy is recommended
> - Most of the evidence for pharmacotherapy is in small numbers of patients over short time frames and this cannot be used to justify maintenance pharmacotherapy
> - Use of pharmacotherapy follows similar approaches to those of mental state disorders, although the caveats of personality disorder need to be remembered
> - No medication is licensed for use in personality pathology

10.1 Summary to personality disorder pharmacotherapy

Although the evidence for the use of medication in personality disorder is minimal, it is increasing. There is no evidence for polypharmacy and most, if not all, prescribing is off-licence (also known as off-label). The strongest evidence for prescribing is for patients with borderline personality disorder for whom mood stabilizers and second-generation antipsychotics (SGAs) may be helpful. Weaker evidence also exists for the use of selective serotonin re-uptake inhibitors (SSRIs) in these patients. The use of antipsychotics in patients with cluster A personality disorders may be of benefit. Presence of a personality disorder is in no way a contraindication to treatment of mental state disorder, but practical considerations, such as an increased risk of overdose, may need to be considered.

Patients with personality pathology, particularly if cared for in secondary services, are invariably treated with pharmacotherapy. Often a number of trials of treatment occur and there may be a natural unwillingness on the part of the physician to stop medication if there is some suggestion of improvement during such a trial. It is often difficult to know if improvements are related to the effects of a drug, particularly bearing in mind the waxing and waning nature of personality problems, and this is a constant clinical challenge. Many patients ultimately take polypharmacy in a stable fashion, although at this point there is no evidence to recommend this or facilitate decision making. Despite this there is a growing research base on the use of pharmacotherapy for personality problems, and this evidence base is largely with regard to borderline personality disorder. It is possible that this disorder has garnered the most interest as it is people with these disorders who routinely present asking for help, rather than patients with schizoid, anxious, or avoidant personality problems. This treatment-seeking group, the borderline group, are those for whom the most evidence exists and they are the patients primarily discussed in this chapter unless otherwise stated.

10.2 General principles of pharmacotherapy for personality disorders

When considering medication use for personality disorder, a number of general considerations should be borne in mind. These are similar to general prescribing principles. Possibly the most important aspect of prescribing is an awareness of the limitations associated with it. Usually other treatment strategies, such as evidence-based psychotherapy (see Chapter 11), should be considered first. Medication should only be used occasionally and polypharmacy (often the rule rather than the exception) should be avoided if possible.

With respect to prescribing, it is critical to ensure that the patient is an active decision maker, a full participant in the process of deciding to take a drug, understanding the effects, and the duration of any trial. As the evidence base is weak and there are generally a number of drug choices, the doctor is at liberty to offer a number of possibilities. Due to the paucity of evidence regarding its effectiveness, it is not appropriate to insist on pharmacotherapy if a patient does not wish it, albeit that its use may be legally insisted upon under the auspices of mental health legislation. By ensuring the patient is actively involved in the process of deciding on treatment, the responsibility for prescribing is shared and the potential for the patient to use the medication as a device for dividing opinion within the team is minimized. It may also improve adherence and make the process of withdrawing any failure of treatment less difficult from the patient's perspective. Similarly the use of any medication in personality disorder is off-licence and the reasons for the trial should be clear to the patient prior to starting treatment. All medication trials should be considered as an '$n = 1$' trial. After the decision is made to trial a medication, the length of the trial should be made explicit, with appropriate review. The duration of the trial depends on both the disorder itself and the medication. Usually a longer time frame is recommended—8–12 weeks is optimal—to assess fully the medication's objective benefits in light of other fluctuations that may occur. Booking in regular reviews should be part of the initial prescribing routine. For each medication trial it is also important that there be an agreed and written set of measures to assess success. These may be emotional (such as feeling calmer, or being less angry) and behavioural (such as less self-harm by cutting, or less accident and emergency presentations), and be jointly decided by patient and clinician. At the point of review, an assessment as to the effectiveness of the drug needs to be undertaken, using the agreed measures, side-effect profile, and safety assessment. All medication has the potential to be used in overdose and poor adherence, leading to 'hoarding' the medication (or overdosing on the medication) may assist in a decision as to whether to continue or not. Dispensing weekly (or possibly even more frequently than this) minimizes this risk and may allow for a reasonable treatment trial at a reasonable dose if there is some evidence that the chosen medication is having a beneficial effect despite these concerns. Should it be decided to continue medication at the completion of any trial period, the ongoing effectiveness of treatment needs to be assessed regularly. It is clear that personality disorder evolves, and for this reason alone it is unlikely medication used solely to assist with management of personality disorder will continue to have a static beneficial effect indefinitely. It is worth noting that recent national guidelines do not recommend the use of pharmacotherapy in BPD as first line treatment or for extended periods of time.

10.3 Treatment of comorbidity

As discussed in Chapter 13, the comorbidity between mental state disorder and personality disorder is significant and the possibility it exists needs to be carefully assessed. Many mental state disorders are appropriately treated with a variety of medication and the presence of personality pathology may modulate the choice of treatment but does not preclude it. The length of time used to assess medication success may need to be lengthened and adherence to a drug regimen more closely monitored as personality disorder may negatively influence pharmacotherapy for mental state disorder. Evidence also suggests that for many mental state disorders outcomes are poorer in the presence of personality dysfunction and measuring success needs to bear this in mind. In fact some authors have suggested that the 'treatment resistance' encountered in some mental state disorder is more appropriately considered as untreated personality pathology.

10.4 **Use of antidepressant medication**

Antidepressant medications are natural compounds to consider trialling bearing in mind the negative affective state associated with personality disorder and the potential biological underpinnings related to serotonergic pathways. The comorbidity with depressive and anxiety disorders implies a shared neurobiological basis and it has been posited that they share neurobiological dysfunction. Trials with older tricyclic antidepressants to relieve personality symptomatology were not particularly successful. Due to the cardiac risk associated with this class of drug in overdose it is not recommended that they be prescribed if personality pathology is present, except in exceptional circumstances. Although similar trials with monoamine oxidase inhibitors had more positive results, these drugs are rarely used in current psychiatric practice, and are potentially lethal in overdose, again limiting their applicability in a clinical setting. In contrast to this, selective serotonin re-uptake inhibitors (SSRIs) have been shown to be effective for a variety of personality traits and self-harming behaviours. Verkes and colleagues identified a link between paroxetine and reductions in self-harming behaviours, and similar reductions in impulsive aggression, anger, and low mood have been found by other researchers with fluoxetine. These studies are, however, small and their findings should be treated with caution. It is not clear at the current time that any particular SSRI is superior to any other in this group of patients. Similarly, researchers have found small symptomatic trait improvements, rather than resolution of disorder. Antidepressants are, perhaps, best thought of as assisting with specific trait symptom amelioration within any particular personality disorder cluster, rather than good at treating the disorder itself. They are only of definite benefit for depressive symptoms. This is somewhat different from their use in mental state disorder, where evidence is usually diagnosis-based. The use of meta-analysis to improve research findings in part overcomes the problem of small trials; however, trial heterogeneity makes combining these studies problematic. Adding to the difficulties in interpreting meta-analyses (and some primary research) is the exclusion of patients with comorbidity, further limiting the capacity to generalize. For these reasons, the positive benefits of the SSRIs from these clinical trials should be interpreted with caution.

10.5 **Use of antipsychotic medication**

Antipsychotic medications have also been trialled for their effects, largely in borderline personality disorder and schizotypal personality disorder. Bearing in mind similar methodological caveats to those for antidepressant medication, these trials have also shown positive outcomes, with reductions in psychotic-like symptoms as the primary outcome for many. Second-generation antipsychotics are better evidence-based than the older, more potent dopaminergic compounds. There is a natural logic to the use of antipsychotic medication in schizotypal PD with some of the biological evidence suggesting it is more closely aligned with the psychotic disorders. This group of patients benefits from antipsychotics and thus there may be some validity to the claim that patients with schizotypy will benefit similarly. Trials with thiothixene show no benefit, whereas haloperidol may lessen hostility and impulsivity. The newer so-called 'second-generation' antipsychotics risperidone, olanzapine, and aripiprazole all have positive findings for psychotic symptoms in patients with personality pathology. Not all studies are, however, positive and continuation studies have often shown little long-term benefit. This suggests that these medications may be of benefit for short-term use only, in order to manage environmental stresses leading to worsening symptoms over the course of days or weeks. The evidence also suggests benefits in affective instability although the findings in suicidal ideation are mixed. A recent review recommends olanzapine, aripiprazole, and haloperidol for specific symptom traits in BPD, but not the use of SSRIs. They may also be of benefit in the initial stages of engagement to manage symptoms while appropriate psychosocial interventions are arranged and negotiated. This will help to contain the likely emotional difficulties experienced in the early stages of treatment, and act as an adjunct to ongoing psychotherapy rather than be the mainstay of treatment.

10.6 Use of anticonvulsants and lithium

Lithium, carbamazepine, sodium valproate, and the newer anticonvulsants have been trialled regarding their impact in patients predominantly with cluster B personality pathology. As early as 1976, Sheard and colleagues examined the impact of lithium in patients with presumed antisocial traits and anticonvulsants have also been trialled. The results of these trials are mixed, at best suggestive of possible benefit and at worse, so limited by design and trial numbers that the results cannot be generalized to clinical populations. Lithium has not been subjected to rigorous randomized controlled trials (RCT) in personality pathology, although is licensed in the UK for 'aggressive and self-mutilating behaviour'. The evidence for carbamazepine is negative, although valproate, lamotrigine and topiramate have weakly positive benefits in interpersonal problems and impulsivity. In borderline personality disorder, most guidelines do not recommend the use of these drugs, although under specialist supervision, a trial may be considered appropriate.

10.7 Other medication

Benzodiazepines, naltrexone, venlafaxine, and omega-3 fatty acids are other medications that have either been subjected to a trial of treatment or described as having clinical utility. Trials of omega-3 fatty acids show positive reductions in suicidality although they could not be recommended in routine clinical practice at this stage. As yet there is no evidence to support the use of these other medications, and they should be avoided currently as part of routine intervention.

Key references

Cowdry, R. W. Gardner, D. L. Pharmacotherapy of borderline personality disorder: alprazolam, carbamazepine, trifluoperazine, and tranylcypromine. *Archives of General Psychiatry* 1988; 45(2): 111.

Goldberg, S. C., Schulz, C. S., Schulz, P. M., Resnick, R. J., Hamer, R. M., Friedel, R. O. Borderline and schizotypal personality disorders treated with low-dose thiothixene vs placebo. *Archives of General Psychiatry* 1986; 43(7): 680–6.

Hallahan, B., Hibbeln, J. R., Davis, J. M., Garland, M. R. Omega-3 fatty acid supplementation in patients with recurrent self-harm Single-centre double-blind randomised controlled trial. *The British Journal of Psychiatry* 2007; 190(2): 118–22.

NICE. *Borderline personality disorder, treatment and management.* London: NICE, 2009.

Verkes, R. J., Van der Mast, R. C., Hengeveld, M. W., Tuyl, J. P., Zwinderman, A. H., Van Kempen, G. M. J. Reduction by paroxetine of suicidal behavior in patients with repeated suicide attempts but not major depression. *American Journal of Psychiatry* 155.4 (1998): 543–7.

Zanarini, M. C., Frankenburg, F. R. Olanzapine treatment of female borderline personality disorder patients: a double-blind, placebo-controlled pilot study. *Journal of Clinical Psychiatry* 2001; 62:849–54.

Chapter 11

Psychotherapy for personality disorder

> **Key points**
> - Psychotherapy is considered to be the first-line strategy for the treatment of personality disorder, although it has evidence only in borderline personality disorder
> - There are now a number of evidence-based psychotherapies for the management of borderline personality disorder

11.1 Summary of personality disorder psychotherapy

Numerous structured therapies have now been developed for the treatment of personality disorder and psychotherapy is seen as the most appropriate modality when considering management options. Dialectical behaviour therapy, mentalization-based therapy, cognitive behaviour therapy for personality disorder, transference focused psychotherapy, cognitive analytical therapy, and systems training for emotional predictability and problem solving are all commonly used evidence-based interventions. Referring patients with personality disorder to a service with a clear evidence-based theoretical approach, with motivated therapists and leaders, is likely to engender clinical benefit, regardless of the specifics of the program.

Although significant progress made over the last two decades reflects the success of clinical researchers, there is little agreement as to the fundamental problems associated with personality dysfunction. This leads to many theoretical approaches being accepted, with different understandings of the underlying issues and diverse ways of addressing these. Adding to the problem is the breadth of diagnostic formulation that constitutes personality disorder, with little agreement about how to diagnose most appropriately in the clinical setting, nor how to ensure uniformity in diagnostic characteristics. Unlike testing the efficacy of a tablet, where the intervention is always the same, the quality of therapy delivered is affected by the leadership of the team, resourcing, seniority of the therapists, and adherence to a specific model. Trials examining a model of therapy developed by a team itself usually outperform real-world trials and they can be considered 'proof of theory' trials rather than effectiveness trials. This said, there is now a significant number of RCTs examining the effectiveness of therapy in personality disorder. The most extensively studied is dialectical behaviour therapy (DBT) for borderline personality disorder (BPD); however, mentalization-based treatment (MBT), cognitive behavioural therapy for personality disorder, transference-focused psychotherapy, cognitive analytical therapy, schema-focused therapy, and systemic training for emotional predictability and problem solving are all evidence-based in RCTs.

11.2 **Similarities in approaches to borderline personality disorder**

Although therapies have different theoretical backgrounds, each has surprisingly similar outcomes in terms of the effect sizes. This raises questions about whether the general similarities between each therapy are more important than the specific interventions each entails. This is the case in general psychotherapy, where nonspecific common factors are excellent predictors of positive outcome. Each successful therapeutic approach is structured, with active therapists who are focused on the relational aspects of the interaction. There is a focus on a strong working alliance and empathy with a clear acknowledgment of the need to take a problem-solving approach. Directly identifying risky behaviours, acknowledging and addressing them as a priority is another common theme. It is likely that these factors enable the patient to feel safe and work on managing his or her own problems as well as providing containment for therapists when working with these clients. Both MBT and DBT add to this by supporting the therapists directly, in order to address and manage counter-transference issues.

11.3 **Dialectical behavioural therapy**

DBT is successfully implemented around the world, leading to a significant volume of research, Internet sites, training centres as well as various manuals and books for patients and DBT clinicians. This heuristic suggests that DBT is the best treatment for personality disorder and is the modality the clinician is most likely to be presented with when considering treatment options for a patient with personality disorder. In one of the first of the explanatory papers, DBT is identified as a cognitive therapy for repeated self-harm, the self-harm seen as a coping mechanism for intolerable psychic distress. DBT has been repeatedly proven effective for women who self-harm irrespective of diagnosis and many of these people will have personality disorder, notably borderline personality disorder. DBT essentially blends a combination of cognitive and behavioural approaches (such as diary cards, skills training, and chain analysis) with self-regulation (mindfulness) in order to allow patients to improve recognition and regulation of their emotional tone. The aim is to improve mindfulness, interpersonal effectiveness, emotion regulation, and distress tolerance. This process, broadly developed though a four-stage approach, seeks to reduce symptom distress and improve subjective quality of life. Reduction of life-threatening behaviours (NSSI) is a key early strategy. DBT is a therapeutic process that usually takes a year, occasionally more, with a combination of individual and group therapy and 'consult groups' for the therapists to attend. The thirteen RCTs examining the effectiveness of DBT leave little doubt that compared to treatment as usual (TAU), DBT is effective at reducing self-harming behaviours and time spent in hospital. It is less clear that DBT is cost effective or improves overall quality of life although there is some evidence of improved social functioning. Qualitative research identifies that patients see the relational aspect of therapy with their individual therapist as key, with the ability to hold the 'dialectic' between acceptance and change as conducive to positive progress. The importance of equality and effective skills training (a CBT-based skill) is also highlighted.

11.4 **Mentalization-based treatment**

Although having a psychodynamic basis, MBT shares many elements of DBT. It eschews interpretations, instead aiming to increase mentalization skills of each patient. It is based on the concept of a failure in attachment development leading to a failure as an adult to understand one's own and others' mental states. The therapy developed from this is designed to improve self-reflection and occurs both through individual therapy as well as group analytic therapy, expressive therapy, and community meetings. Through therapy, patients develop the capacity to manage emotional regulation and consider outcomes prior to acting. Initially MBT was developed to be delivered using partial hospitalization, although this has recently been trialled in an outpatient setting. Eight-year follow-up of this group shows sustained improvements and this compares highly favourably to the six to eight week trials of medication.

11.5 Other cognitive and behavioural therapies

These therapies (CBT-PD, STEPPS, and SFT) are based on the structured approach to psychotherapy focused on developing connections between a patient's thoughts, feelings, and behaviour. Although CBT was initially formulated for depressive disorders, it has been modified to be applied to personality problems. The emphasis of therapy has moved towards an understanding of historical experiences that lead to the dysfunctional thoughts that drive feelings. These are used to experience and understand current problems with the development of behavioural interventions and cognitive process in order to improve emotional and interpersonal skills. SFT explores the development of dysfunctional cognitive schema and uses limited re-parenting to address these in therapy. More pragmatic approaches have modified CBT for application by those with a general mental health background, increasing applicability in a public mental health setting. CBT-PD focuses on the relational aspects of therapy, with structured and collaborative formulation as its cornerstone. CBT-PD is one of the few therapies to be trialled in the community for patients with personality disorder other than BPD, with some benefit. STEPPS is a group therapy designed to address emotional regulation in a structured way. Importantly these CBT-based approaches show reductions in self-harm.

11.6 Other analytically based therapies

Rather than the basic assumptions made by cognitive and behaviour therapies, an alternative view suggests that the development of personality dysfunction is related to damaged psychodynamic development variously thought of as being due to a lack of capacity to attach, disturbed internalized object relations, or a lack of a developed personal identity. Such theoretical underpinning leads to a different style of therapy, aimed at allowing the patient to develop internal constructs which will help him or her manage interactions with the world better. There is little or no focus on specific skills training; instead, the focus is on understanding the self and the self in relationship to others. Transference-focused psychotherapy (TFT) is a manualized form of analytic therapy of benefit in BPD. Therapy occurs twice a week in an individualized format, with a focus on interpreting transference in order to allow the patient to reactivate internalized object relations. The comparative paper by Clarkin and colleagues (2004) is one of the few RCTs to compare formal therapy for personality disorder (in this case BPD) from different modalities. They compared TFT with DBT and supportive treatment over a one-year period. Using a growth curve analysis, they posit benefits of TFT over the other two modalities. Although this trial has not been replicated it emphasizes the importance of relational input. Cognitive analytic therapy (CAT) applies object relations theory to patients in order to allow them to form a greater understanding of self, and it included elements of cognitive therapy. As with CBT-PD it is time-limited and designed to allow patients to improve their understanding of relational problems. It has been shown to be effective in adolescents with BPD, although not currently so in the adults.

11.7 **Therapeutic communities**

Historically, therapeutic communities have been developed to allow a safe space for patients with personality problems to recover. The emphasis is on relationships both with the therapist and with others in the community as the key elements to the process of growth in personality, aiming to strengthen positive emotional and interpersonal responses. Therapeutic communities (TC) have a structured theoretical approach and clear principles by which to operate. Traditional TCs are becoming increasingly rare; the costs associated with them are making them unsustainable. This has led to the development of TCs that do not require a full-time residential setting and in some cases they now occur online.

Key references

Bateman, A., Fonagy, P. 8-year follow-up of patients treated for borderline personality disorder: mentalization-based treatment versus treatment as usual. *American Journal of Psychiatry* 2008; 165(5): 631–8.

Chanen, A. M., Jackson, H. J., McCutcheon, L. K., Jovev, M., Dudgeon, P., Yuen, H. P., Germano, D., Nistico, H., McDougall, E., Weinstein, C., Clarkson, V., McGorry, P. D. Early intervention for adolescents with borderline personality disorder using cognitive analytic therapy: randomised controlled trial. *British Journal of Psychiatry* 2008; 193(6): 477–84.

Clarkin, J.F., Levy, K.N., Lenzenweger, M.F., Kernberg, O.F. The Personality Disorders Institute/Borderline Personality Disorder Research Foundation Randomized Control Trial for Borderline Personality Disorder: Rationale, Methods, and Patient Characteristics. *Journal of Personality Disorders* 2004; 18(1): 52–72.

Cunningham, K., Wolbert, R., Lillie, B. It's about me solving my problems: Clients' assessments of dialectical behavior therapy. *Cognitive and Behavioral Practice* 2004; 11(2): 248–56.

Kendall, T., Pilling, S., Tyrer, P., Duggan, C., Burbeck, R., Meader, N., Taylor, C. Guidelines: Borderline and Antisocial Personality Disorders: Summary of NICE Guidance. *British Medical Journal* 2009; 338 (7689): 293–5.

Kernberg, O. Borderline personality organization. *Journal of the American Psychoanalytic Association* 1967; 15(3): 641–85.

Marsha M. Linehan, M. M. Dialectical Behavioral Therapy: A Cognitive Behavioral Approach to Parasuicide. Journal of Personality Disorders: 1987; 1(4): 328–33.

Messer, S. B., Wampold, B. E. Let's face facts: Common factors are more potent than specific therapy ingredients. *Clinical Psychology: Science and Practice* 2002; 9(1): 21–5.

Öst, L-G. Efficacy of the third wave of behavioral therapies: A systematic review and meta-analysis. *Behaviour research and therapy* 2008; 46(3): 296–321.

Chapter 12

Other interventions and strategies in the management of personality disorder

> **Key points**
>
> - There are multiple approaches to supporting patients with personality problems, and a lack of evidence is not the same as evidence of no effect
> - Pragmatic approaches, such as education and practical support, should not be overlooked
> - Alternative therapies and novel approaches may be of benefit, depending on individual circumstance
> - A best-fit approach between patient and intervention is clinically sensible

57

12.1 Summary of alternative interventions and management of personality disorder

Although the evidence for pharmacotherapy and psychotherapy is now established, this does not mean a variety of other approaches may not be sensible for individual patients. A lack of evidence to support an intervention is not the same as evidence of ineffective treatment. Consideration of alternative strategies to express and understand emotion, such as art or drama therapy, may be beneficial. There is some evidence that environmental change and nido-therapy may offer novel approaches to patients who have difficulties in finding a fit between themselves and their environment.

A variety of alternative, complementary, and other therapies have been used and trialled in attempts to assist people with difficulties in managing themselves and their relationships with others. These therapists often specifically identify personality disturbance, and occasionally describe its general features, if not diagnosing personality disorder specifically. Much of the management of personality disturbance occurs outside a medical or psychiatric setting and, particularly in milder forms, this is potentially both appropriate as treatment and a better use of resources. Although many of these other forms of management are not evidence-based, this does not mean that they are unhelpful or that they do not work. It means that they fall outside the evidence-based medicine paradigm and this fact needs to be taken into account. A values-based-medicine approach captures these more fully and may be a better paradigm to work within when considering complex disorders and complex management strategies for them.

12.2 Psycho-education and family support

The need to support families has already been discussed (see Chapters 5–7), and undertaking this in a structured way can be useful. Being clear about diagnosis, particularly in terms of what this means with regard to management, and prognosis can help family to conceptualize the problems facing their family member and support him or her during times of emotional dysfunction, anxiety, withdrawal, or despair. Numerous books for the layperson have now been published, outlining some of the difficulties facing patients in a straightforward manner. Realizing 'it's not just happening to us' can be a major relief to families, friends, and the patients themselves. Indeed, whole networks now exist with the purpose of supporting families who struggle with personality disorder, particularly borderline personality disorder. These networks recognize the difficulties for the entire family, and take a whole-system approach to supporting the patient. Much of this input does not require direct medical supervision, but being able to identify the family's need for help and direct patients to such networks can be highly valuable.

12.3 **Art therapies**

Art therapies have been used in psychiatry for decades and are routinely used in the management of personality disorder in some areas. Art therapy, movement therapy, and music therapy each involve the application of creative skills and talents to express the self in a safe environment. These expressions can then be used to provide context for patients to understand their internal world. Often art therapies are used as part of a complex structured intervention for patients with personality disorder and although these interventions have their use, the impact of the art therapy itself is not well established. Patients describe the process as useful and one which allows them to communicate their difficulties in a non-verbal way.

12.4 **Nidotherapy**

Nidotherapy is a new structured therapy designed for patients with severe and enduring mental disorders, the overwhelming proportion of whom have personality pathology comorbid with mental state disorder. This form of therapy assumes that the patient's mental disorder is largely intractable and it endeavours to work with the patient through a nidotherapist to alter the environment instead the personality. This approach is quite different from more traditional management strategies as its primary focus is environmental-based rather than patient-based change. There is limited evidence that this form of therapy may be of benefit, and its evaluation remains in the very early stages.

12.5 **The 'best fit' approach**

In all alternative therapies and more mainstream approaches the notion of 'best fit' remains important. The relational aspects of therapy are essential and even in behavioural 'here and now' therapies or the provision of medication, the capacity to acknowledge, accept, and work as equals in the patient–therapist relationships adds value. Understanding the nature of this relationship is perhaps the key element in the management of personality pathology and a common element across all effective psychotherapies and alternative therapies. The ability to develop rapport and trust, manage distress, and tolerate difference marks out the successful therapist. When considering the possibility of complementary therapies, an awareness of the patient's strengths may lead to a recommendation of the use of such an approach prior to the instigation of a more structured, formal, talking therapy. Although all patients with personality disorder share certain elements of distress, each is unique and requires an individualized and flexible approach.

Key references

Crawford, M., Rutter, D., Price, K., Weaver, T., Josson, M., Tyrer, P., Gibson, S., Gillespie, S., Faulkner, A., Ryrie, I., Dhillon, K., Bateman, A., Fonagy, P. Taylor, B., Moran, P., Beckett, J., Blackwell, H., Burbridge, C., Coldham, T., Gould, D., Imlack, S., Parfoot, S., Sheldon, K., Sweeney, A., Taylor, E.Learning the lessons: A multi-method evaluation of dedicated community-based services for people with personality disorder. Report for the National Co-ordinating Centre for NHS Service Delivery and Organisation R&D (NCCSDO) 2007: 191.

Newton-Howes, G., Weaver, P., Tyrer, P. Attitudes of staff towards patients with personality disorder in community mental health teams. *Australian and New Zealand Journal of Psychiatry* 2008: 42(7): 572–7.

Porr, V. *Overcoming Borderline Personality Disorder: A Family Guide for Healing and Change.* Oxford: Oxford University Press, 2010.

Chapter 13

The impact of personality pathology on mental state disorders

Key points

- Personality pathology alters the presentation and prognosis of mental state disorders
- Often this comorbidity leads to 'treatment resistance', or residual symptomatology that requires management consideration
- More aggressive treatment of mental state disorder may be necessary in the presence of personality disorder

13.1 Summary of the impact on mental state disorders of personality pathology

Personality disorder comorbid with mental state disorder presents challenges to secondary care services and this comorbidity is increasingly likely as the overall severity of psychopathology present increases. In depressive disorders, personality disorder worsens both initial presentation and prognosis, although aggressive treatment of the depression may ameliorate this effect. Anxiety disorders have considerable overlap with cluster C personality pathology, although early studies suggested poorer outcome, later studies are more equivocal. The research into personality in bipolar and psychotic disorders is less well developed, although in both mental state disorders personality can be teased out to be a focus of future research. Personality disorder is present in more than half of all patients with substance-use disorders and has been a focus of clinical trials, although this remains at the research stage.

Understanding how to recognize personality pathology, formulating personality difficulties, and developing a management strategy are all essential clinical tools; however, the presentation of personality disorder in a general psychiatric setting is often coloured by the presence of comorbid mental state disorder. Indeed it is often the failure to manage a complex depression or similar mental state problem adequately that initiates a referral to psychiatric services from primary care. There is some postulation that these referrals or treatment-resistant presentations may in fact be due to unrecognized personality problems rather than attributable to a true failure to respond to treatment for mental state disorder. Disentangling mental state disorders from personality disorder is complex, primarily as many symptoms can be common to both, but it is possible to do this clinically. This chapter reviews how the presence of personality pathology influences the course of various mental state disorders but does not directly address the question of coordinated treatment. This is a growing and complex field which remains in its infancy. Because it is developing quickly, referral to local specialist personality disorder services is usually appropriate.

13.2 **Depressive disorders**

Significant work has been done on the impact of personality disorder and dysfunction in the presence of depressive disorders, with many depression trials examining the impact of personality on outcome. Comorbidity is high with as many as 100 per cent of depressed patients fulfilling the criteria for a personality disorder at some time. Test–re-test research identifies that the identification of personality problems in clinically depressed patients is possible, although it is potentially difficult. Many of the arguments about the reliability of the personality diagnosis in this cohort simply reflect the difficulties of personality disorder diagnosis in both clinical practice and the research setting (see Chapter 4). Although any personality disorder can be present, the most commonly found categories include avoidant/anxious/dependent personalities (the fearful group), but borderline personality disorder and personality disorder NOS also feature prominently. Although the literature is mixed, it appears that comorbidity worsens the prognosis with respect to recovery from depressive disorders. Personality pathology affects both symptom domains and social functioning in a negative way. The deterioration in prognosis is as much as a doubling in the resistance to treatment for depression. This would suggest aggressive management of depression in the presence of personality pathology is warranted. Identification of personality pathology should also lead to a consideration of what, if any, additional management strategies may be helpful and allows for increased prognostic clarity.

13.3 **Anxiety disorders**

The similarities between anxiety disorders (generalized anxiety disorder, panic disorder with/without agoraphobia, social phobia, and obsessive–compulsive disorder), and anxious–avoidant personality disorders have been noted in terms of the diagnostic symptoms and, when the longitudinal course is taken into account (both are chronic), a time classifier does not provide for differentiation. Although the genetic data are mixed, there is likely to be a strong a link between trait neuroticism, anxiety disorders, and the serotonin transporter promoter polymorphism 5-HTTLPR. Trait studies, particularly using the five-factor model for neuroticism, are consistent and suggest that this personality trait is also associated with axis I disorder. Studies of categorical personality disorders are somewhat more mixed. Early studies suggest poorer outcomes for the anxiety disorders with comorbid anxious–avoidant personality problems although later studies are more equivocal. It is likely that there is a degree of overlap between these disorders and the association of one to the other in terms of outcome is a factor in this. Personality disorders have been shown to worsen remission from generalized anxiety disorder by almost one-third, with a similar impact in social phobia. Similar results have been found for panic disorder although these findings are less clear. If patients with anxiety disorder are followed up in the long term, there is a strong association between personality disorder and poor social functioning, even if there is apparent symptom remission. This suggests personality dysfunction may comprise the 'treatment resistance' in some anxious patients, rather than it being a core feature of the disorder itself.

13.4 **Bipolar affective disorders**

The potential consanguinity between bipolar affective disorder (BPAD) and borderline personality disorder (BPD) has been the major focus of attention in respect of bipolar mood disorder and personality disorder. Basset's focus on the similarities between the two disorders notes symptomatic similarities including affective dysregulation, depressive features (particularly atypical), self-mutilation, reduced limbic modulation, and disrupted sleep. Despite these numerous similarities he, along with others, recognizes the significant clusters of divergent symptoms and suggests comorbidity but not a spectrum-like disorder. From a treatment perspective, the significantly better outcomes in BPAD with pharmacotherapy and differences in focus of psychotherapy are also important. BPAD patients show sustained improvements with mood-regulating pharmacotherapy and these are beneficial for prophylaxis. This is not the case for BPD where a wide variety of antipsychotics and some mood stabilizers can have predominantly short-term benefits. Most psychotherapies for BPD focus on management of emotional dysregulation whereas BPAD therapy is more actively focused or has a psycho-educational perspective. There is remarkably little research into the influence of BPAD in other personality disorder subtypes. More general personality screening in the presence of bipolarity suggests trait neuroticism predicts a poorer course in BPAD although little further than this can be said. This is not an entirely surprising finding and more focused research is clearly needed.

13.5 Psychotic disorders

One of the initial concepts of psychotic mental disorder was the notion that psychotic phenomena represented the deterioration of personality itself. There is more recent evidence of a biological connection between the odd personality disorders and psychotic mental disorder both biologically (see Chapter 3) and clinically (see Chapter 5), with both potentially lying along the same biological pathway. It may not be sensible, therefore, to think about the odd personality disorders as comorbid with schizophrenia, but instead they may be consanguineous with it. Nonetheless, personality has been assessed in psychosis and a huge variation in prevalence has been reported. This is affected by multiple study variables. What is not clear from the literature is how the presence of personality pathology (schizotypal or other) impacts on schizophrenia management and this is an area that requires further work, particularly bearing in mind the largely cognitive approaches to managing emergent social problems in patients with psychosis, and the generally held belief that these problems are irreversible and largely deteriorate over time.

13.6 Substance-use disorders

The combination of substance-use disorders (SUDS) and personality problems is both obvious and increasingly researched. This research follows two distinct lines: epidemiological research into the comorbidity of substance-use disorders from large scale addictions research, and trials of treatment of substance-use disorders in patients with comorbid personality problems. The evidence for establishing the impact of SUDs on personality disorders or the direct treatment thereof is still emerging. The reasons for the association between SUDs and personality problems is not clear but a number of hypotheses have been made. The most likely hypothesis posits a direct causal link between personality disorder and SUDs, the existence of the former leading to the development of the latter. Other theories include the possibility of one disorder influencing a third variable and this leading to the development of the second relationship (indirect causality), and there being no causal relationship but shared genetic and environmental risk factors that lead to both disorders. The National Epidemiologic Survey on Alcohol and Related Conditions (NESARC) found comorbidity as great as 58 per cent for alcohol use disorders in the presence of borderline personality disorder, and similarly raised rates are found in antisocial personality disorder. Both are externalizing personality disorders and this is where the primary connection appears to lie. In terms of treatment, trials have investigated dialectical behaviour therapy for substance abuse (DBT-S) and dual-focus schema therapy (DFST). These are both essentially cognitive-behaviour models of psychotherapy that aim to improve coping strategies and prevent one or other disorder sabotaging treatment. To-date the trials of these specific treatments do not indicate significant improvements over well-structured routine addictions care; however, these treatment developments are encouraging future directions for management. Consideration has also been given to the possibility of an 'addictive personality', although a comprehensive review of the topic identifies this as unlikely to exist.

Key references

Bassett, D. Borderline personality disorder and bipolar affective disorder. Spectra or spectre? A review. *Australian and New Zealand Journal of psychiatry* 2012; 46(4): 327–39.

Massion, A. O., Dyck, I. R., Shea, M. T., Phillips, K. A. Personality disorders and time to remission in generalized anxiety disorder, social phobia, and panic disorder. *Archives of General Psychiatry* 2002; 59(5): 434.

Mulder, R. T. Alcoholism and personality. *Australian and New Zealand Journal of Psychiatry* 2002; 36(1): 44–52.

Mulder, R. T. Depression and personality disorder. *Current psychiatry reports* 2004; 6(1): 51–7.

Siever, L. J., & Davis, K. L. A psychobiologic perspective on the personality disorders. *American Journal of Psychiatry* 1991; 148: 1647–58.

Chapter 14

Conclusion

The diagnosis, treatment, and management of personality disorder remains a complex, challenging, and important part of psychiatric practice presenting the clinician with numerous difficulties both at the level of basic understanding and clinical application. At one end of the spectrum, personality is considered a normal part of the human condition, studied in order to be understood but lying outside the realms of psychiatry. At the other end, its existence potentially explains a significant proportion of the psychiatric and social morbidity in the community and the 'treatment resistance' of mental state disorder. This view places personality disorder at the forefront of need for evaluation and treatment. Experts in personality pathology from across disciplines agree that personality disorder is both important and requires further understanding but there is little agreement as to how best to even classify personality coherently to permit this, let alone integrate the research conducted to-date. These difficulties at the research level often leave the clinician unsure of the value of a personality disorder diagnosis and this may in part explain the wide variation in the prevalence found between research and clinical populations. The divergence in the direction of classification between DSM-5, which continues to use a system which divides disorders into ten categories, and the possibility of a diagnostic system based on dimensions of disorder and their severity suggested by ICD-11 is a clear example of the difficulties the field is facing.

Having said this, GPs, emergency medicine physicians, and psychiatrists routinely see patients with minimal mental state disorder but significant psychological difficulty. These patients struggle to understand themselves and display disrupted attachment to others. This distress is often acted out leading to harms to the patient, their family, and the wider community. These individuals are personality disordered and they seek support. Others internalize these problems and cause considerable distress to family and friends, although they may not see this. Others still experience repeated conflict in society, and eventually end up in prison or the judicial system. The burden in each case is significant on the person themselves and also on society.

Although work remains to be done in understanding the nature of personality pathology in a way that is both scientifically accurate and clinically applicable, progress has been made in finding therapeutic solutions. Identifying the problems and ruling out mental state disorder prevents poorly rationalized trials of treatment, and starts the process of allowing the patient and family to recognize and understand the issues at hand. Providing a theoretically grounded, consistent therapy via motivated, skilled, and supported therapists gives the patient the emotional space to consider the difficulties he or she is facing within a safe psychological framework, possibly using the relational aspects of therapy to begin the healing process. Review by an expert diagnostician rules out other psychiatric disorder, for which these patients are at greater risk, and allows for the judicious and short-term use of psychotropic medication to support the patient in therapy. Finally, allowing the patient to develop an effective risk plan minimizes the possibility of a serious adverse event occurring, giving time for growth and development, without positively reinforcing potentially destructive behaviours. As further research begins to more accurately clarify the key diagnostic issues, treatment will undoubtedly become more targeted. Right now however, adhering to these principles provides a sound framework for the patient to begin to get better and for the therapist to feel safe and confident in clinical practice.

Key reference

Bernstein, D. P., Iscan, C. Maser, J. Opinions of personality disorder experts regarding the DSM-IV personality disorders classification system. *Journal of Personality Disorders* 2007; 21(5): 536–51.

Index

67